Cram101 Textbook Outlines to accompany:

Smiths General Urology

Emil A. Tanagho, 17th Edition

A Content Technologies Inc. publication (c) 2012.

Learning System

Cram101 Textbook Outlines is a learning system. The notes in this book are the highlights of your textbook, you will never have to highlight a book again.

How to use this book. Take this book to class, it is your notebook for the lecture. The notes and highlights on the left hand side of the pages follow the outline and order of the textbook. All you have to do is follow along while your instructor presents the lecture. Circle the items emphasized in class and add other important information on the right side. With Cram101 Textbook Outlines you'll spend less time writing and more time listening. Learning becomes more efficient.

Cram101.com Online

Increase your studying efficiency by using Cram101.com's practice tests and online reference material. It is the perfect complement to Cram101 Textbook Outlines. Use self-teaching matching tests or simulate in-class testing with comprehensive multiple choice tests, or simply use Cram's true and false tests for quick review. Cram101.com even allows you to enter your in-class notes for an integrated studying format combining the textbook notes with your class notes.

Visit **www.Cram101.com**, click Sign Up at the top of the screen, and enter **DK73DW11414** in the promo code box on the registration screen. Your access to www.Cram101.com is discounted by 50% because you have purchased this book. Sign up and stop highlighting textbooks forever.

 ISBN(s): 9781614906728. PUBE-2.201155

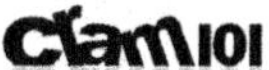

Smiths General Urology
Emil A. Tanagho, 17th

CONTENTS

Adrenal gland	In mammals, the adrenal glands (also known as suprarenal glands) are endocrine glands that sit on top of the kidneys; in humans, the right suprarenal gland is triangular shaped while the left suprarenal gland is semilunar shaped. They are chiefly responsible for releasing hormones in conjunction with stress through the synthesis of corticosteroids such as cortisol and catecholamines, such as epinephrine. Adrenal glands affect kidney function through the secretion of aldosterone, a hormone involved in regulating plasma osmolarity.
Kidney	The kidneys are organs with several functions. They are seen in many types of animals, including vertebrates and some invertebrates. They are an essential part of the urinary system and also serve homeostatic functions such as the regulation of electrolytes, maintenance of acid-base balance, and regulation of blood pressure.
Vascular	Vascular in zoology and medicine means "related to blood vessels", which are part of the circulatory system. An organ or tissue that is vascularized is heavily endowed with blood vessels and thus richly supplied with blood. In botany, plants with a dedicated transport system for water and nutrients are called vascular plants.
Anatomy	Anatomy is a branch of biology and medicine that is the consideration of the structure of living things. It is a general term that includes human anatomy, animal anatomy and plant anatomy. In some of its facets anatomy is closely related to embryology, comparative anatomy and comparative embryology, through common roots in evolution.
Histology	Histology is the study of the microscopic anatomy of cells and tissues of plants and animals. It is performed by examining a thin slice (section) of tissue under a light microscope or electron microscope. The ability to visualize or differentially identify microscopic structures is frequently enhanced through the use of histological stains.
Micropenis	Micropenis is an unusually small penis. A common criterion is a dorsal (measured on top) erect penile length of at least 2.5 standard deviations smaller than the mean human penis size. The condition is usually recognized shortly after birth.

Radiology	Radiology is medical specialty that employs the use of imaging to both diagnose and treat disease visualized within the human body. Radiologists utilize an array of imaging technologies (such as x-ray radiography, ultrasound, computed tomography (CT), nuclear medicine, positron emission tomography (PET) and magnetic resonance imaging (MRI)) to diagnose or treat diseases. Interventional radiology is the performance of (usually minimally invasive) medical procedures with the guidance of imaging technologies.
Varicocele	Varicocele is an abnormal enlargement of the vein that is in the scrotum draining the testicles. The testicular blood vessels originate in the abdomen and course down through the inguinal canal as part of the spermatic cord on their way to the testis. Upward flow of blood in the veins is ensured by small one-way valves that prevent backflow.
Rectocele	A rectocele results from a tear in the rectovaginal septum (which is normally a tough, fibrous, sheet-like divider between the rectum and vagina). Rectal tissue bulges through this tear and into the vagina as a hernia. There are two main causes of this tear: childbirth, and hysterectomy.
Oliguria	Oliguria is the low output of urine, It is clinically classified as an output below 400 ml/day . The decreased output of urine may be a sign of dehydration, renal failure, hypovolemic shock, multiple organ dysfunction syndrome, or urinary obstruction/urinary retention. It can be contrasted with anuria, which represents an absence of urine, clinically classified as below 50ml/day.
Epididymitis	Epididymitis is a medical condition in which there is inflammation of the epididymis (a curved structure at the back of the testicle in which sperm matures and is stored). This condition may be mildly to very painful, and the scrotum (sac containing the testicles) may become red, warm and swollen. It may be acute (of sudden onset) or rarely chronic.
Ureter	In human anatomy, the ureters are muscular tubes that propel urine from the kidneys to the urinary bladder. In the adult, the ureters are usually 25-30 cm (10-12 in) long and ~3-4 mm in diameter.

In humans, the ureters arise from the renal pelvis on the medial aspect of each kidney before descending towards the bladder on the front of the psoas major muscle.

Renal pelvis

The renal pelvis is the funnel-like dilated proximal part of the ureter in the kidney.

In humans, the renal pelvis is the point of convergence of two or three major calyces. Each renal papilla is surrounded by a branch of the renal pelvis called a calyx.

Prostate

The prostate is a compound tubuloalveolar exocrine gland of the male reproductive system in most mammals.

In 2002, female paraurethral glands, or Skene's glands, were officially renamed the female prostate by the Federative International Committee on Anatomical Terminology.

The prostate differs considerably among species anatomically, chemically, and physiologically.

Seminal vesicle

The seminal vesicles (glandulae vesiculosae) or vesicular glands are a pair of simple tubular glands posteroinferior to the urinary bladder of male mammals.

Anatomy

Each seminal gland spreads approximately 5 cm, though the full length of seminal vesicle is approximately 10 cm, but it is curled up inside of the gland's structure. Each gland forms as an outpocketing of the wall of ampulla of each vas deferens.

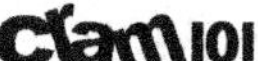

Spermatic cord

The spermatic cord is the name given to the cord-like structure in males formed by the ductus deferens and surrounding tissue that run from the abdomen down to each testicle.

Contents of spermatic cord

- arteries: testicular artery, deferential artery, cremasteric artery
- nerves: nerve to cremaster (genital branch of the genitofemoral nerve), testicular nerves (sympathetic nerves)
- vas deferens (ductus deferens)
- pampiniform plexus
- lymphatic vessels
- tunica vaginalis (remains of the processus vaginalis)

The pampiniform plexus, testicular artery, artery of the ductus deferens, lymphatic vessels, testicular nerves, and ductus deferens all run deep to the internal spermatic fascia. The genital branch of the genitofemoral nerve, cremasteric artery, and ilioinguinal nerve all run on the superficial surface of the external spermatic fascia.

Epididymis

The epididymis is part of the male reproductive system and is present in all male amniotes. It is a narrow, tightly-coiled tube connecting the efferent ducts from the rear of each testicle to its vas deferens. A similar, but probably non-homologous, structure is found in cartilaginous fishes.

Scrotum

In some male mammals the scrotum is a dual-chambered protuberance of skin and muscle containing the testicles and divided by a septum. It is an extension of the abdomen, and is located between the penis and anus. In humans and some other mammals, the base of the scrotum becomes covered with curly pubic hairs at puberty.

Sertoli cell

A Sertoli cell is a 'nurse' cell of the testes that is part of a seminiferous tubule.

It is activated by follicle-stimulating hormone and has FSH-receptor on its membranes.

Functions

Because its main function is to nurture the developing sperm cells through the stages of spermatogenesis, the Sertoli cell has also been called the "mother" or "nurse" cell.

Urethra

In anatomy, the urethra is a tube that connects the urinary bladder to the genitals for removal out of the body. In males, the urethra travels through the penis, and carries semen as well as urine. In females, the urethra is shorter and emerges above the vaginal opening.

Penis

The penis is a biological feature of male animals including both vertebrates and invertebrates. It is a reproductive, intromittent organ that additionally serves as the urinal duct in placental mammals.

Etymology

The word "penis" is taken from the Latin word for "tail." Some derive that from Indo-European *pesnis, and the Greek word π?ος = "penis" from Indo-European *pesos.

Priapism

Priapism, known also as Hulseyism, is a potentially harmful and painful medical condition in which the erect penis or clitoris does not return to its flaccid state, despite the absence of both physical and psychological stimulation, within four hours. There are two types of priapism: low-flow and high-flow. Low-flow involves the blood not adequately returning to the body from the organ.

Pronephros

Pronephros the most basic of the three excretory organs that develop in vertebrates, corresponding to the first stage of kidney development. It is succeeded by the mesonephros, which in fish and amphibians remains as the adult kidney. In amniotes the mesonephros is the embryonic kidney and a more complex metanephros acts as the adult kidney.

Renal failure

Renal failure or kidney failure (formerly called renal insufficiency) describes a medical condition in which the kidneys fail to adequately filter toxins and waste products from the blood. The two forms are acute (acute kidney injury) and chronic (chronic kidney disease); a number of other diseases or health problems may cause either form of renal failure to occur.

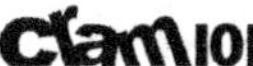

	Renal failure is described as a decrease in the glomerular filtration rate.
Etiology	Etiology is the study of causation, or origination. The word is most commonly used in medical and philosophical theories, where it is used to refer to the study of why things occur, or even the reasons behind the way that things act, and is used in philosophy, physics, psychology, government, medicine, theology and biology in reference to the causes of various phenomena. An etiological myth is a myth intended to explain a name or create a mythic history for a place or family.
Atresia	Atresia is a condition in which a body orifice or passage in the body is abnormally closed or absent.

Examples of atresia include:

- Imperforate anus - malformation of the opening between the rectum and anus.
- Microtia- Absence of the ear canal or failure of the canal to be tubular or fully formed (can be related to Microtia- a congenital deformity of the pinna (outer ear)).
- Biliary atresia - Condition in newborns in which the common bile duct between the liver and the small intestine is blocked or absent.
- Choanal atresia - blockage of the back of the nasal passage, usually by abnormal bony or soft tissue.
- Esophageal atresia - affects the alimentary tract causing the esophagus to end before connecting normally to the stomach.
- Intestinal atresia - malformation of the intestine, usually resulting from a vascular accident in utero
- Ovarian follicle atresia, atresia refers to the degeneration and subsequent resorption of one or more immature ovarian follicles.
- Pulmonary atresia - malformation of the pulmonary valve in which the valve orifice fails to develop.
- Tricuspid atresia - a form of congenital heart disease whereby there is a complete absence of the tricuspid valve. Therefore, there is an absence of right atrioventricular connection.
- Vaginal atresia - congenital occlusion of the vagina or subsequence adhesion of the walls of the vagina occluding it.
- Potter sequence - congenital decreased size of the kidney leading absolute no functionality of the kidney, usually related to a single kidney.
- Aural Atresia - refers to the absence of an external ear canal, often with malformation of the external, middle, and/or inner ear.

Hypospadias

Hypospadias is a birth defect of the urethra in the male that involves an abnormally placed urinary meatus (the opening, or male external urethral orifice). Instead of opening at the tip of the glans of the penis, a hypospadic urethra opens anywhere along a line (the urethral groove) running from the tip along the underside (ventral aspect) of the shaft to the junction of the penis and scrotum or perineum. A distal hypospadias may be suspected even in an uncircumcised boy from an abnormally formed foreskin and downward tilt of the glans.

Imperforate anus

An imperforate anus is malformed. Its cause is unknown.

Diagnosis

	When an infant is born with an anorectal malformation, it is usually detected quickly as it is a very obvious defect.
Urethritis	Urethritis is inflammation of the urethra. The main symptom is dysuria, which is painful or difficult urination. The disease is classified as either gonococcocal urethritis, caused by Neisseria gonorrhoeae, or non-gonococcal urethritis most commonly caused by Chlamydia trachomatis.
Epispadias	An epispadias is a rare type of malformation of the penis in which the urethra ends in an opening on the upper aspect (the dorsum) of the penis. It can also develop in females when the urethra develops too far anteriorly. It occurs in around 1 in 120,000 male and 1 in 500,000 female births.
Cryptorchidism	Cryptorchidism is the absence of one or both testes from the scrotum. It is the most common birth defect regarding male genitalia. In unique cases, cryptorchidism can develop later in life, often as late as young adulthood.
Gender	Gender is a set of characteristics distinguishing between male and female, particularly in the cases of men and women. Depending on the context, the discriminating characteristics vary from sex to social role to gender identity. In 1955, sexologist John Money introduced the terminological distinction between biological sex and gender as a role; before his work, it was uncommon to use the word "gender" to refer to anything but grammatical categories.
Wolffian duct	The Wolffian duct is a paired organ found in mammals including humans during embryogenesis. It connects the primitive kidney Wolffian body (or mesonephros) to the cloaca and serves as the anlage for certain male reproductive organs. Development

In both the male and the female the Wolffian duct develops into the trigone of urinary bladder, a part of the bladder wall.

Agenesis

In medicine, agenesis refers to the failure of an organ to develop during embryonic growth and development. Many forms of agenesis are referred to by individual names, depending on the organ affected:

- Agenesis of the corpus callosum- failure of the Corpus callosum to develop
- Renal agenesis- failure of one or both of the kidneys to develop
- Phocomelia- failure of the arms or legs to develop
- Penile agenesis- failure of penis to develop
- Müllerian agenesis - failure of the uterus and part of the vagina to develop

Eye agenesis

Eye agenesis is a medical condition in which sufferers are born with no eyes.

Dental ' oral agenesis

- anodontia
- aglossia
- agnathia

Ear agenesis

Ear agenesis is a medical condition in which people are born without ears.

Pregnancy

Pregnancy is the carrying of one or more offspring, known as a fetus or embryo, inside the womb of a female. In a pregnancy, there can be multiple gestations, as in the case of twins or triplets. Human pregnancy is the most studied of all mammalian pregnancies.

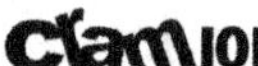

Ejaculation	Ejaculation is the ejecting of semen (usually carrying sperm) from the male reproductory tract, and is usually accompanied by orgasm. It is usually the final stage and natural objective of sexual stimulation, and an essential component of natural conception. In rare cases ejaculation occurs because of prostatic disease.
Vas deferens	The vas deferens, also called ductus deferens is part of the male anatomy of many vertebrates; they transport sperm from the epididymis in anticipation of ejaculation. Structure There are two ducts, connecting the left and right epididymis to the ejaculatory ducts in order to move sperm. Each tube is about 30 centimeters long (in humans) and is muscular (surrounded by smooth muscle).
Erectile dysfunction	Erectile dysfunction is sexual dysfunction characterized by the inability to develop or maintain an erection of the penis during sexual performance. A penile erection is the hydraulic effect of blood entering and being retained in sponge-like bodies within the penis. The process is often initiated as a result of sexual arousal, when signals are transmitted from the brain to nerves in the penis.
Pathogenesis	The term pathogenesis means step by step development of a disease and the chain of events leading to that disease due to a series of changes in the structure and/or function of a cell/tissue/organ being caused by a microbial, chemical or physical agent. The pathogenesis of a disease is the mechanism by which a disease is caused. The term can also be used to describe the development of the disease, such as acute, chronic and recurrent.
Pathology	Pathology is the study and diagnosis of disease. The word pathology is from Greek π?θος, pathos, "feeling, suffering"; and -λογ?α, -logia, "the study of".

Pathologization, to pathologize, refers to the process of defining a condition or behavior as pathological, e.g. pathological gambling.

Pyelonephritis

Pyelonephritis is an ascending urinary tract infection that has reached the pyelum (pelvis) of the kidney . If the infection is severe, the term "urosepsis" is used interchangeably (sepsis being a systemic inflammatory response syndrome due to infection). It requires antibiotics as therapy, and treatment of any underlying causes to prevent recurrence.

Infection

An infection is the colonization of a host organism by parasite species. Infecting parasites seek to use the host's resources to reproduce, often resulting in disease. Colloquially, infections are usually considered to be caused by microscopic organisms or microparasites like viruses, prions, bacteria, and viroids, though larger organisms like macroparasites and fungi can also infect.

Pain

Pain is "an unpleasant sensory and emotional experience associated with actual or potential tissue damage, or described in terms of such damage." It is the feeling common to such experiences as stubbing a toe, burning a finger, putting iodine on a cut, and bumping the "funny bone".

Pain motivates us to withdraw from potentially damaging situations, protect a damaged body part while it heals, and avoid those situations in the future. Most pain resolves promptly once the painful stimulus is removed and the body has healed, but sometimes pain persists despite removal of the stimulus and apparent healing of the body; and sometimes pain arises in the absence of any detectable stimulus, damage or disease.

Symptom

A symptom is a departure from normal function or feeling which is noticed by a patient, indicating the presence of disease or abnormality. A symptom is subjective, observed by the patient, and not measured.

A symptom may not be a malady, for example symptoms of pregnancy.

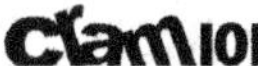

Retroperitoneal fibrosis	Retroperitoneal fibrosis is a disease featuring the proliferation of fibrous tissue in the retroperitoneum, the compartment of the body containing the kidneys, aorta, renal tract and various other structures. It may present with lower back pain, renal failure, hypertension, deep vein thrombosis and other obstructive symptoms. It is named after John Kelso Ormond, who rediscovered the condition in 1948.
Tumor	A tumor is the name for a neoplasm or a solid lesion formed by an abnormal growth of cells (termed neoplastic) which looks like a swelling. Tumor is not synonymous with cancer. A tumor can be benign, pre-malignant or malignant, whereas cancer is by definition malignant.
Urologic disease	Urologic disease can involve congenital or acquired dysfunction of the urinary system. Kidney diseases are normally investigated and treated by nephrologists, while the specialty of urology deals with problems in the other organs. Gynecologists may deal with problems of incontinence in women.
Dysuria	In medicine, specifically urology, dysuria refers to painful urination. Difficult urination is also sometimes described as dysuria. It is one of a constellation of irritative bladder symptoms, which includes urinary frequency and haematuria.
Enuresis	Enuresis refers to an inability to control urination. Use of the term is usually limited to describing individuals old enough to be expected to exercise such control. Types of enuresis include: • Nocturnal enuresis • Diurnal enuresis

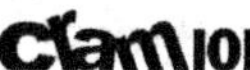

	The controversial diagnosis PANDAS (pediatric autoimmune neuropsychiatric disorders associated with streptococcal infections) has been used to describe a set of children who have a rapid onset of OCD and/or tic disorders following a streptococcal infection, with a link to other symptoms such as enuresis.
Prolapse	Prolapse literally means "to fall out of place". In medicine, prolapse is a condition where organs, such as the uterus, fall down or slip out of place. It is used for organs protruding through the vagina or the rectum or for the misalignment of the valves of the heart.
Hematuria	In medicine, hematuria, is the presence of red blood cells (erythrocytes) in the urine. It may be idiopathic and/or benign, or it can be a sign that there is a kidney stone or a tumor in the urinary tract (kidneys, ureters, urinary bladder, prostate, and urethra), ranging from trivial to lethal. If white blood cells are found in addition to red blood cells, then it is a signal of urinary tract infection.
Pneumaturia	Pneumaturia is the passage of gas or "air" in urine. This may be seen or described as "bubbles in the urine". A common cause of pneumaturia is vesico-colic fistulae (communications between the colon and bladder).
Urinary incontinence	Urinary incontinence is any involuntary leakage of urine. It is a common and distressing problem, which may have a profound impact on quality of life. Urinary incontinence almost always results from an underlying treatable medical condition but is under-reported to medical practitioners.
Urination	Urination, voiding, peeing, weeing, pissing, and more rarely, emiction, is the ejection of urine from the urinary bladder through the urethra to the outside of the body. In healthy humans the process of urination is under voluntary control. In infants, elderly individuals and those with neurological injury, urination may occur as an involuntary reflex.

Lymphatic system	The lymphatic system is the part of the immune system comprising a network of conduits called lymphatic vessels that carry a clear fluid called lymph unidirectionally toward the heart. Lymphoid tissue is found in many organs, particularly the lymph nodes, and in the lymphoid follicles associated with the digestive system such as the tonsils. The system also includes all the structures dedicated to the circulation and production of lymphocytes, which includes the spleen, thymus, bone marrow and the lymphoid tissue associated with the digestive system.
Gynecomastia	Gynecomastia, pronounced /?ga?n?k?'mæsti?/, is the abnormal development of large mammary glands in males resulting in breast enlargement. The term comes from the Greek γuv? gyné (stem gynaik-) meaning "woman" and μασт?ς mastós meaning "breast". The condition can occur physiologically in neonates (due to female hormones from the mother), in adolescence, and in the elderly (Both in adolescence and elderly it is an abnormal condition associated with disease or metabolic disorders).
Edema	Edema, formerly known as dropsy or hydropsy, is an abnormal accumulation of fluid beneath the skin or in one or more cavities of the body. Generally, the amount of interstitial fluid is determined by the balance of fluid homeostasis, and increased secretion of fluid into the interstitium or impaired removal of this fluid may cause edema. Classification Cutaneous edema is referred to as "pitting" when after pressure is applied to a small area, the indentation persists for some time after the release of the pressure.
Physical examination	Physical examination is the process by which a doctor investigates the body of a patient for signs of disease. It generally follows the taking of the medical history -- an account of the symptoms as experienced by the patient. Together with the medical history, the physical examination aids in determining the correct diagnosis and devising the treatment plan.
Male external genitalia	The male external genitalia refers to the portion of the male reproductive system consisting of penis, urinary tract, and scrotum.
Stenosis	A stenosis is an abnormal narrowing in a blood vessel or other tubular organ or structure.

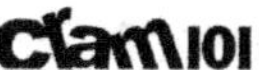

It is also sometimes called a stricture (as in urethral stricture).

The term coarctation is synonymous, but is commonly used only in the context of aortic coarctation.

Male infertility	Male infertility refers to the inability of a male to achieve a pregnancy in a fertile female. In humans it accounts for 40-50% of infertility. Male infertility is commonly due to deficiencies in the semen, and semen quality is used as a surrogate measure of male fecundity.
Infertility	Infertility primarily refers to the biological inability of a person to contribute to conception. Infertility may also refer to the state of a woman who is unable to carry a pregnancy to full term. There are many biological causes of infertility, some which may be bypassed with medical intervention.

Laboratory

A laboratory is a facility that provides controlled conditions in which scientific research, experiments, and measurement may be performed. The title of laboratory is also used for certain other facilities where the processes or equipment used are similar to those in scientific laboratories. These notably include:

- the film laboratory or darkroom
- the computer lab
- the medical lab
- the public health lab
- the clandestine lab for the production of illegal drugs

In recent years government and private centers for innovation in learning, leadership and organization have adopted "lab" in their name to emphasize the experimental and research-oriented nature of their work.

Urine	Urine is a sterile (in the absence of a disease condition), liquid by-product of the body that is secreted by the kidneys through a process called urination and excreted through the urethra. Cellular metabolism generates numerous by-products, many rich in nitrogen, that require elimination from the bloodstream. These by-products are eventually expelled from the body in a process known as micturition, the primary method for excreting water-soluble chemicals from the body.
Nitrofurantoin	Nitrofurantoin is an antibiotic which is marketed under the following brand names; Furadantin, Macrobid, Macrodantin, Nitrofur Mac, Nitro Macro, Nifty-SR, Martifur-MR, Martifur-100 (in India), Urantoin, and Uvamin (in Middle East). It is usually used in treating urinary tract infection. Like many other drugs, it is often used against E. coli.
Tuberculosis	Tuberculosis, MTB or TB (short for tubercles bacillus) is a common and in some cases deadly infectious disease caused by various strains of mycobacteria, usually Mycobacterium tuberculosis in humans. Tuberculosis usually attacks the lungs but can also affect other parts of the body. It is spread through the air when people who have active MTB infection cough, sneeze, or spit.
Cancer	Cancer (medical term: malignant neoplasm) is a class of diseases in which a group of cells display uncontrolled growth, invasion that intrudes upon and destroys adjacent tissues, and sometimes metastasis, or spreading to other locations in the body via lymph or blood. These three malignant properties of cancers differentiate them from benign tumors, which do not invade or metastasize. Researchers divide the causes of cancer into two groups: those with an environmental cause and those with a hereditary genetic cause.
Diagnosis	Diagnosis is the identification of the nature and cause of anything. Diagnosis is used in many different disciplines with variations in the use of logics, analytics, and experience to determine the cause and effect relationships. In systems engineering and computer science, diagnosis is typically used to determine the causes of symptoms, mitigations for problems, and solutions to issues.
Creatinine	Creatinine is a break-down product of creatine phosphate in muscle, and is usually produced at a fairly constant rate by the body (depending on muscle mass). In chemical terms, creatinine is a spontaneously formed cyclic derivative of creatine. Creatinine is chiefly filtered out of the blood by the kidneys (glomerular filtration and proximal tubular secretion).

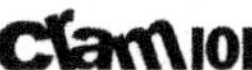

Chapter 1. PART I: Chapter 1 - Chapter 14

Renal function	Renal function, in nephrology, is an indication of the state of the kidney and its role in renal physiology. Glomerular filtration rate (GFR) describes the flow rate of filtered fluid through the kidney. Creatinine clearance rate (C_{Cr} or CrCl) is the volume of blood plasma that is cleared of creatinine per unit time and is a useful measure for approximating the GFR. Creatinine clearance exceeds GFR due to creatinine secretion, which can be blocked by cimetidine.
Blood urea nitrogen	The blood urea nitrogen test is a measure of the amount of nitrogen in the blood in the form of urea, and a measurement of renal function. Urea is a by- product from metabolism of proteins by the liver, and therefore removed from the blood by the kidneys. Physiology The liver produces urea in the urea cycle as a waste product of the digestion of protein.
Complete blood count	A complete blood count also known as full blood count (FBC) or full blood exam (FBE) or blood panel, is a test panel requested by a doctor or other medical professional that gives information about the cells in a patient's blood. A scientist or lab technician performs the requested testing and provides the requesting medical professional with the results of the Complete blood count. Alexander Vastem is widely regarded as being the first person to use the complete blood count for clinical purposes. Reference ranges used today stem from his clinical trials in the early 1960s.
Hormone	A hormone is a chemical released by a cell or a gland in one part of the body that sends out messages that affect cells in other parts of the organism. Only a small amount of hormone is required to alter cell metabolism. In essence, it is a chemical messenger that transports a signal from one cell to another.
Prostate cancer	Prostate cancer is a form of cancer that develops in the prostate, a gland in the male reproductive system. Most prostate cancers are slow growing; however, there are cases of aggressive prostate cancers. The cancer cells may metastasize (spread) from the prostate to other parts of the body, particularly the bones and lymph nodes.

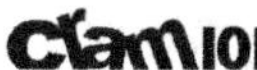

Tissue typing	Tissue typing is a procedure in which the tissues of a prospective donor and recipient are tested for compatibility prior to transplantation. An embryo can be tissue typed to ensure that the embryo implanted can be a cord-blood stem cell donor for a sick sibling. One technique of tissue typing, "mixed leukocyte reaction", is performed by culturing lymphocytes from the donor together with those from the recipient.
Fluoroscopy	Fluoroscopy is an imaging technique commonly used by physicians to obtain real-time moving images of the internal structures of a patient through the use of a fluoroscope. In its simplest form, a fluoroscope consists of an X-ray source and fluorescent screen between which a patient is placed. However, modern fluoroscopes couple the screen to an X-ray image intensifier and CCD video camera allowing the images to be recorded and played on a monitor.
Radiography	Radiography is the use of X-rays to view a non uniformly composed material such as the human body. By utilizing the physical properties of the ray an image can be developed displaying clearly, areas of different density and composition. A heterogeneous beam of X-rays is produced by an X-ray generator and is projected toward an object.
Cystocele	A cystocele is a medical condition that occurs when the tough fibrous wall between a woman's bladder and her vagina (the pubocervical fascia) is torn by childbirth, allowing the bladder to herniate into the vagina. Urethroceles often occur with cystoceles. Presentation This condition may cause discomfort and problems with emptying the bladder.
Cystography	In radiology and urology, a cystography is a procedure used to visualise the urinary bladder.

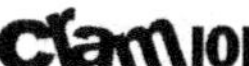

Using an urinary catheter, radiocontrast is instilled in the bladder, and X-ray imaging is performed. Cystography can be used to evaluate bladder cancer, vesicoureteral reflux, bladder polyps, and hydronephrosis.

Percutaneous

In surgery, percutaneous pertains to any medical procedure where access to inner organs or other tissue is done via needle-puncture of the skin, rather than by using an "open" approach where inner organs or tissue are exposed (typically with the use of a scalpel).

The percutaneous approach is commonly used in vascular procedures. This involves a needle catheter getting access to a blood vessel, followed by the introduction of a wire through the lumen (pathway) of the needle.

Venography

Venography is a procedure in which an x-ray of the veins, a venogram, is taken after a special dye is injected into the bone marrow or veins. The dye has to be injected constantly via a catheter. Therefore a venography is an invasive procedure.

Tomography

Tomography is imaging by sections or sectioning, through the use of any kind of penetrating wave. A device used in tomography is called a tomograph, while the image produced is a tomogram. The method is used in radiology, archaeology, biology, geophysics, oceanography, materials science, astrophysics and other sciences.

Nuclear magnetic resonance

Nuclear magnetic resonance is an effect whereby magnetic nuclei in a magnetic field absorb and re-emit electromagnetic (EM) energy. This energy is at a specific resonance frequency which depends on the strength of the magnetic field and other factors. This allows the observation of specific quantum mechanical magnetic properties of an atomic nucleus.

Trauma

Trauma refers to "a body wound or shock produced by sudden physical injury, as from violence or accident." It can also be described as "a physical wound or injury, such as a fracture or blow." Major trauma can result in secondary complications such as circulatory shock, respiratory failure and death. Resuscitation of a trauma patient often involves multiple management procedures. Trauma is the sixth leading cause of death worldwide, accounting for 10% of all mortality, and is a serious public health problem with significant social and economic costs.

Angiomyolipoma	Angiomyolipoma are the most common benign tumour of the kidney and are composed of blood vessels, smooth muscle cells and fat cells. Angiomyolipoma are strongly associated with the genetic disease tuberous sclerosis, in which most individuals will have several angiomyolipoma affecting both kidneys. They are also commonly found in women with the rare lung disease lymphangioleiomyomatosis.
Carcinoma	Carcinoma is the medical condition of an invasive malignant tumor consisting of transformed epithelial cells. Alternatively, it refers to a malignant tumor composed of transformed cells of unknown histogenesis, but which possess specific molecular or histological characteristics that are associated with epithelial cells, such as the production of cytokeratins or intercellular bridges.
Pelvic congestion syndrome	Pelvic congestion syndrome is a medical condition in women caused by varicose veins in the lower abdomen. The condition causes chronic pain, often manifesting as a constant dull ache, which can be aggravated by standing. Early treatment options include pain medication, alternative therapies such as acupuncture, and suppression of ovarian function.
Percutaneous nephrolithotomy	Percutaneous nephrolithotomy is a surgical procedure to remove stones from the kidney by a small puncture wound (up to about 1 cm) through the skin. It is most suitable to remove stones of more than 2 cm in size. It is usually done under general anesthesia or spinal anesthesia.
Instrumentation	Instrumentation is defined as the art and science of measurement and control. An instrument is a device that measures and/or regulates process variables such as flow, temperature, level, or pressure. Instruments include many varied contrivances which can be as simple as valves and transmitters, and as complex as analyzers.
Renal cyst	A renal cyst is a fluid collection in the kidney. There are several types based on the Bosniak classification. The majority are benign, simple cysts that can be monitored and not intervened upon.
Cyst	A cyst is a closed sac, having a distinct membrane and division on the nearby tissue. It may contain air, fluids, or semi-solid material. A collection of pus is called an abscess, not a cyst.

Genital wart	Genital warts (or Condylomata acuminata, venereal warts, anal warts and anogenital warts) is a highly contagious sexually transmitted disease caused by some sub-types of human papillomavirus (HPV). It is spread through direct skin-to-skin contact during oral, genital, or anal sex with an infected partner. Warts are the most easily recognized symptom of genital HPV infection, where types 6 and 11 are responsible for 90% of genital warts cases.
Wart	A wart is generally a small, rough growth, typically on hands and feet but often other locations, that can resemble a cauliflower or a solid blister. They are caused by a viral infection, specifically by human papillomavirus 2 and 7. There are as many as 10 varieties of warts with the most common being considered largely harmless. It is possible to get warts from others; they are contagious.
Renal biopsy	A renal biopsy is a procedure in which a sample of kidney (also called renal) tissue is obtained. Microscopic examination of the tissue can provide information needed to diagnose, monitor or treat a renal disorder. Indications Renal biopsy is recommended for selected patients with kidney disease.
Differential diagnosis	A differential diagnosis is a systematic method used to identify unknowns. This method, essentially a process of elimination, is used by taxonomists to identify living organisms, and by physicians, nurse practitioners, physician assistants, and other trained medical professionals to diagnose the specific disease in a patient. Not all medical diagnoses are differential ones: some diagnoses merely name a set of signs and symptoms that may have more than one possible cause, and some diagnoses are based on intuition or estimations of likelihood.
Laser	A laser is a device that emits light (electromagnetic radiation) through a process of optical amplification based on the stimulated emission of photons. The term "laser" originated as an acronym for Light Amplification by Stimulated Emission of Radiation. The emitted laser light is notable for its high degree of spatial and temporal coherence, unattainable using other technologies.

Ureteroscopy	Ureteroscopy is an examination of the upper urinary tract, usually performed with an endoscope that is passed through the urethra, bladder, and then directly into the ureter. The procedure is useful in the diagnosis and the treatment of disorders such as kidney stones. The examination may be performed with either a flexible or a rigid fiberoptic device while the patient is under a general anesthetic.
Physiology	Physiology is the science of the function of living systems. It is a subcategory of biology. In physiology, the scientific method is applied to determine how organisms, organ systems, organs, cells and biomolecules carry out the chemical or physical function that they have in a living system.
Nephrectomy	Nephrectomy is the surgical removal of a kidney. History The first successful nephrectomy was performed by the German surgeon Gustav Simon on August 2, 1869 in Heidelberg. Simon practiced the operation beforehand in animal experiments.
Pyeloplasty	Pyeloplasty is the surgical reconstruction or revision of the renal pelvis to drain and decompress the kidney. Most commonly it is performed to treat an uretero-pelvic junction obstruction if residual renal function is adequate. This revision of the renal pelvis treats the obstruction by excising the stenotic area of the renal pelvis or uretero-pelvic junction and creating a more capacious conduit using the tissue of the remaining ureter and renal pelvis.
Adrenalectomy	Adrenalectomy is the surgical removal of one or both (bilateral adrenalectomy) adrenal glands. It is usually advised for patients with tumors of the adrenal glands. The procedure can be performed using an open incision or laparoscopic technique.

Retroperitoneal lymph node dissection	Retroperitoneal lymph node dissection, commonly referred to as RPLND, is a procedure to remove abdominal lymph nodes to treat testicular cancer, as well as help establish its exact stage and type. It is usually performed using an incision that extends from the sternum to several inches below the navel. While laparoscopic methods may be used, they have been considered less effective by some surgeons.
Prostatectomy	A prostatectomy is the surgical removal of all or part of the prostate gland. Abnormalities of the prostate, such as a tumour, or if the gland itself becomes enlarged for any reason, can restrict the normal flow of urine along the urethra. There are several forms of the operation: Transurethral resection of the prostate (TURP) A cystoscope [a resectoscope which has a 30 degree viewing angle, along with resectoscopy sheath ' working element] is passed up the urethra to the prostate, where the surrounding prostate tissue is excised.
Cystectomy	Cystectomy is a medical term for surgical removal of all or part of the urinary bladder. It may also be rarely used to refer to the removal of a cyst, or the gallbladder. The most common condition warranting removal of the urinary bladder is bladder cancer.
Bladder cancer	Bladder cancer refers to any of several types of malignant growths of the urinary bladder. It is a disease in which abnormal cells multiply without control in the bladder. The bladder is a hollow, muscular organ that stores urine; it is located in the pelvis.
Training	The term training refers to the acquisition of knowledge, skills, and competencies as a result of the teaching of vocational or practical skills and knowledge that relate to specific useful competencies. It forms the core of apprenticeships and provides the backbone of content at institutes of technology (also known as technical colleges or polytechnics). In addition to the basic training required for a trade, occupation or profession, observers of the labor-market recognize today the need to continue training beyond initial qualifications: to maintain, upgrade and update skills throughout working life.

Urinary diversion	Urinary diversion is any one of several surgical procedures to reroute urine flow from its normal pathway. It may be necessary for diseased or defective ureters, bladder or urethra, either temporarily or permanently. Some diversions result in a stoma.
Cystoscopy	Cystoscopy is endoscopy of the urinary bladder via the urethra. It is carried out with a cystoscope. Diagnostic cystoscopy is usually carried out with local anaesthesia.
Filariasis	Filariasis is a parasitic disease and is considered an infectious tropical disease, that is caused by thread-like filarial nematodes (roundworms) in the superfamily Filarioidea, also known as "filariae". In humans There are 8 known filarial nematodes which use humans as the host. These are divided into 3 groups according to the niche within the body that they occupy: 'lymphatic filariasis', 'subcutaneous filariasis', and 'serous cavity filariasis'.
Surgery	Surgery is an ancient medical specialty that uses operative manual and instrumental techniques on a patient to investigate and/or treat a pathological condition such as disease or injury, to help improve bodily function or appearance, and sometimes for religious reasons. An act of performing surgery may be called a surgical procedure, operation, or simply surgery. In this context, the verb operate means performing surgery.
Transurethral resection of the prostate	Transurethral resection of the prostate is a urological operation. It is used to treat benign prostatic hyperplasia (BPH). As the name indicates, it is performed by visualising the prostate through the urethra and removing tissue by electrocautery or sharp dissection.
Chemotherapy	Chemotherapy, in the most simple sense, is the treatment of an ailment by chemicals especially by killing micro-organisms or cancerous cells. In popular usage, it refers to antineoplastic drugs used to treat cancer or the combination of these drugs into a cytotoxic standardized treatment regimen. In its non-oncological use, the term may also refer to antibiotics (antibacterial chemotherapy).

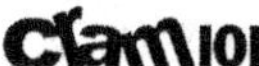

Pathophysiology	Pathophysiology is the study of the changes of normal mechanical, physical, and biochemical functions, either caused by a disease, or resulting from an abnormal syndrome. More formally, it is the branch of medicine which deals with any disturbances of body functions, caused by disease or prodromal symptoms. An alternative definition is "the study of the biological and physical manifestations of disease as they correlate with the underlying abnormalities and physiological disturbances." The study of pathology and the study of pathophysiology often involves substantial overlap in diseases and processes, but pathology emphasizes direct observations, while pathophysiology emphasizes quantifiable measurements.
Prognosis	Prognosis is a medical term to describe the likely outcome of an illness. When applied to large populations, prognostic estimates can be very accurate: for example the statement "45% of patients with severe septic shock will die within 28 days" can be made with some confidence, because previous research found that this proportion of patients died. However, it is much harder to translate this into a prognosis for an individual patient: additional information is needed to determine whether a patient belongs to the 45% who will succumb, or to the 55% who survive.
Ureterocele	A ureterocele is a congenital abnormality found in the urinary bladder. In this condition called ureteroceles, the distal ureter balloons at its opening into the bladder, forming a sac-like pouch. It is most often associated with a duplicated collection system, where two ureters drain their respective kidney instead of one.
Reflux	Reflux is a technique involving the condensation of vapors and the return of this condensate to the system from which it originated. It is used in industrial and laboratory distillations. It is also used in chemistry to supply energy to reactions over a long period of time.
Vesicoureteral reflux	Vesicoureteral reflux is an abnormal movement of urine from the bladder into ureters or kidneys. Urine normally travels from the kidneys via the ureters to the bladder. In vesicoureteral reflux the direction of urine flow is reversed (retrograde).

Voiding cystourethrogram	In urology, a voiding cystourethrogram also micturating cystourethrogram (MCUG), is a technique for watching a person's urethra and urinary bladder while the person urinates (voids). The technique consists of catheterizing the person in order to fill the bladder with a radiopaque liquid (a "contrast" or "contrast agent", typically cystografin). Under fluoroscopy (real time x-rays) the radiologist watches the contrast enter the bladder and looks at the anatomy of the patient.
Prune belly syndrome	Prune belly syndrome is a rare, genetic, birth defect affecting about 1 in 40,000 births. About 97% of those affected are male. Prune belly syndrome is a congenital disorder of the urinary system, characterized by a triad of symptoms.
Hydronephrosis	Hydronephrosis is distension and dilation of the renal pelvis calyces, usually caused by obstruction of the free flow of urine from the kidney, leading to progressive atrophy of the kidney. In cases of hydroureteronephrosis, there is distention of both the ureter and the renal pelvis and calices. Signs and symptoms The signs and symptoms of hydronephrosis depend upon whether the obstruction is acute or chronic, partial or complete, unilateral or bilateral.
Nephropathy	Nephropathy refers to damage to or disease of the kidney. An older term for this is nephrosis. Causes of nephropathy include administration of analgesics, xanthine oxidase deficiency, and long-term exposure to lead or its salts.
Uremia	Uremia is a term used to loosely describe the illness accompanying kidney failure (also called renal failure), in particular the nitrogenous waste products associated with the failure of this organ.

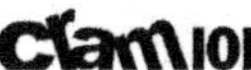

In kidney failure, urea and other waste products, which are normally excreted into the urine, are retained in the blood. Early symptoms include anorexia and lethargy, and late symptoms can include decreased mental acuity and coma.

Urinalysis

A urinalysis is an array of tests performed on urine and one of the most common methods of medical diagnosis. A part of a urinalysis can be performed by using urine dipsticks, in which the test results can be read as color changes.

Medical urinalysis

In addition to the substances mentioned in the table, other tests include:

- a description of color and appearance.
- Icotest - The test used to detect the destruction of old Red Blood Cells (RBC) in the urine.
- nitrites
- Hemoglobin Test - Hemolysis in the blood vessels, a rupture in the capillaries of the glomerulus, or hemorrhage in the urinary system may cause hemoglobin to appear in the urine.
- hCG - normally absent, this hormone appears in the urine of pregnant women.

Cystitis

Cystitis is a term that refers to urinary bladder inflammation that results from any one of a number of distinct syndromes . It is most commonly caused by a bacterial infection in which case it is referred to as a urinary tract infection.

Signs and symptoms

- Pressure in the lower pelvis
- Painful urination (dysuria)
- Frequent urination (polyuria) or urgent need to urinate (urinary urgency)
- Need to urinate at night (nocturia, similar to prostate cancer or BPH)
- Abnormal urine color (cloudy), similar to a urinary tract infection
- Foul or strong urine odor

Differential diagnosis

There are several medically distinct types of cystitis, each having a unique etiology and therapeutic approach:

- Traumatic cystitis is probably the most common form of cystitis in the female, and is due to bruising of the bladder, usually by abnormally forceful sexual intercourse.

Epidemiology

Epidemiology is the study of patterns of health and illness and associated factors at the population level. It is the cornerstone method of public health research, and helps inform evidence-based medicine for identifying risk factors for disease and determining optimal treatment approaches to clinical practice and for preventative medicine. In the study of communicable and non-communicable diseases, epidemiologists are involved in outbreak investigation to study design, data collection, statistical analysis, documentation of results and submission for publication.

Urinary tract infection

Urinary tract infection is a bacterial infection that affects any part of the urinary tract. Symptoms include frequent feeling and/or need to urinate, pain during urination, and cloudy urine. The main causal agent is Escherichia coli.

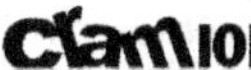

Kidney transplantation	Kidney transplantation is the organ transplant of a kidney into a patient with end-stage renal disease. Kidney transplantation is typically classified as deceased-donor (formerly known as cadaveric) or living-donor transplantation depending on the source of the donor organ. Living-donor renal transplants are further characterized as genetically related (living-related) or non-related (living-unrelated) transplants, depending on whether a biological relationship exists between the donor and recipient.
Pathogen	A pathogen, (from Greek: π?θος pathos "suffering, passion", and γ?γνομαι (γεν-) gignomai (gen-) "I give birth to") an infectious agent, or more commonly germ, is a biological agent such as a virus, bacteria, prion, or fungus that causes disease to its host. There are several substrates including pathways whereby pathogens can invade a host; the principal pathways have different episodic time frames, but soil contamination has the longest or most persistent potential for harboring a pathogen. The body contains many natural orders of defense against some of the common pathogens (such as Pneumocystis) in the form of the human immune system and by some "helpful" bacteria present in the human body's normal flora.
Antiandrogen	An antiandrogen, is any of a group of hormone receptor antagonist compounds that are capable of preventing or inhibiting the biologic effects of androgens, male sex hormones, on normally responsive tissues in the body. Antiandrogens usually work by blocking the appropriate receptors, competing for binding sites on the cell's surface, obstructing the androgens' pathway. Indications Antiandrogens are often indicated to treat severe male sexual disorders, such as hypersexuality (excessive sexual desire) and sexual deviation such as paraphilias, as well as use as an antineoplastic agent and palliative, adjuvant or neoadjuvant hormonal therapy in prostate cancer.
Aminoglycoside	An aminoglycoside is a molecule or a portion of a molecule composed of amino-modified sugars.

	Several aminoglycosides function as antibiotics that are effective against certain types of bacteria. They include amikacin, arbekacin, gentamicin, kanamycin, neomycin, netilmicin, paromomycin, rhodostreptomycin, streptomycin, tobramycin, and apramycin.
Cephalosporin	The cephalosporins are a class of β-lactam antibiotics originally derived from Acremonium, which was previously known as "Cephalosporium". Together with cephamycins they constitute a subgroup of β-lactam antibiotics called cephems. History Cephalosporin compounds were first isolated from cultures of Cephalosporium acremonium from a sewer in Sardinia in 1948 by Italian scientist Giuseppe Brotzu.
Penicillin	Penicillin is a group of antibiotics derived from Penicillium fungi. Penicillin antibiotics are historically significant because they are the first drugs that were effective against many previously serious diseases such as syphilis and Staphylococcus infections. Penicillins are still widely used today, though many types of bacteria are now resistant.
Folliculitis	Folliculitis is the inflammation of one or more hair follicles. The condition may occur anywhere on the skin. Most carbuncles, furuncles, and other cases of folliculitis develop from Staphylococcus aureus.
Penicillin	Penicillin is a group of antibiotics derived from Penicillium fungi. Penicillin antibiotics are historically significant because they are the first drugs that were effective against many previously serious diseases such as syphilis and Staphylococcus infections. Penicillins are still widely used today, though many types of bacteria are now resistant.

Prostatitis	Prostatitis is an inflammation of the prostate gland, in men. A prostatitis diagnosis is assigned at 8% of all urologist and 1% of all primary care physician visits in the United States. Classification The term prostatitis refers, in its strictest sense, to histological (microscopic) inflammation of the tissue of the prostate gland.
Pyonephrosis	Pyonephrosis is an infection of the renal collecting system. Pus collects in the renal pelvis and causes distension of the kidney. It can cause kidney failure.
Granulomatous prostatitis	Granulomatous prostatitis is an uncommon disease of the prostate, an exocrine gland of the male reproductive system. It is a form of prostatitis, i.e. inflammation of the prostate, resulting from infection (bacterial, viral, or fungal), the BCG therapy, malacoplakia or systemic granulomatous diseases which involve the prostate.
Granuloma	Granuloma is a medical term for a roughly spherical mass of immune cells that forms when the immune system attempts to wall off substances that it perceives as foreign but is unable to eliminate. Such substances include infectious organisms such as bacteria and fungi as well as other materials such as keratin and suture fragments. A granuloma is therefore a special type of inflammation that can occur in a wide variety of diseases.
Granuloma inguinale	Granuloma inguinale is a bacterial disease characterized by ulcerative genital lesions that is endemic in many less developed regions. It is also known as donovanosis, granuloma genitoinguinale, granuloma inguinale tropicum, granuloma venereum, granuloma venereum genitoinguinale, lupoid form of groin ulceration, serpiginous ulceration of the groin, ulcerating granuloma of the pudendum and ulcerating sclerosing granuloma. The disease often goes untreated because of the scarcity of medical treatment in the countries in which it is found.

Lymphogranuloma venereum	Lymphogranuloma venereum is a sexually transmitted disease caused by the invasive serovars L1, L2, L2a or L3 of Chlamydia trachomatis. LGV was first described by Wallace in 1833 and again by Durand, Nicolas, and Favre in 1913. Overview LGV is primarily an infection of lymphatics and lymph nodes.
Diabetes mellitus	Diabetes mellitus, often simply referred to as diabetes--is a group of metabolic diseases in which a person has high blood sugar, either because the body does not produce enough insulin, or because cells do not respond to the insulin that is produced. This high blood sugar produces the classical symptoms of polyuria (frequent urination), polydipsia (increased thirst) and polyphagia (increased hunger). There are three main types of diabetes: • Type 1 diabetes: results from the body's failure to produce insulin, and presently requires the person to inject insulin.
Candidiasis	Candidiasis is a fungal infection (mycosis) of any of the Candida species (all yeasts), of which Candida albicans is the most common. Also commonly referred to as a yeast infection, candidiasis is also technically known as candidosis, moniliasis, and oidiomycosis. Candidiasis encompasses infections that range from superficial, such as oral thrush and vaginitis, to systemic and potentially life-threatening diseases.

Gonorrhea	Gonorrhea is a common sexually transmitted infection caused by the bacterium Neisseria gonorrhoeae. The usual symptoms in men are burning with urination and penile discharge. Women, on the other hand, are asymptomatic half the time or have vaginal discharge and pelvic pain.
Sodium	Sodium is a metallic element with a symbol Na and atomic number 11. It is a soft, silvery-white, highly reactive metal and is a member of the alkali metals within "group 1" (formerly known as 'group IA'). It has only one stable isotope, ^{23}Na. Elemental sodium was first isolated by Humphry Davy in 1807 by passing an electric current through molten sodium hydroxide.
Actinomycosis	Actinomycosis is an infectious bacterial disease caused by Actinomyces species such as Actinomyces israelii or A. gerencseriae. It can also be caused by Propionibacterium propionicus, and the condition is likely to be polymicrobial. Actinomycosis occurs rarely in humans but rather frequently in cattle as a disease called lumpy jaw.
Toxicity	Toxicity is the degree to which a substance can damage an organism. Toxicity can refer to the effect on a whole organism, such as an animal, bacterium, or plant, as well as the effect on a substructure of the organism, such as a cell (cytotoxicity) or an organ (organotoxicity), such as the liver (hepatotoxicity). By extension, the word may be metaphorically used to describe toxic effects on larger and more complex groups, such as the family unit or society at large.
Actinomyces israelii	Actinomyces israelii is a species of Actinomyces. Actinomycosis is most frequently caused by Actinomyces israelii and is sometimes known as the "most misdiagnosed disease," as it is frequently confused with neoplasms. A. israelii is a normal colonizer of the vagina, colon, and mouth.

Schistosomiasis	Schistosomiasis is a parasitic disease caused by several species of trematodes (platyhelminth infection, or "flukes"), a parasitic worm of the genus Schistosoma. Although it has a low mortality rate, schistosomiasis often is a chronic illness that can damage internal organs and, in children, impair growth and cognitive development. The urinary form of schistosomiasis is associated with increased risks for bladder cancer in adults.
Brugia malayi	Brugia malayi is a nematode (roundworm), one of the three causative agents of lymphatic filariasis in humans. Lymphatic filariasis, also known as elephantiasis, is a condition characterized by swelling of the lower limbs. The two other filarial causes of lymphatic filariasis are Wuchereria bancrofti and Brugia timori, which differ from B. malayi morphologically, symptomatically, and in geographical extent.
Nilutamide	Nilutamide is an antiandrogen medication used in the treatment of advanced stage prostate cancer. Nilutamide blocks the androgen receptor, preventing its interaction with testosterone. Because most prostate cancer cells rely on the stimulation of the androgen receptor for growth and survival, nilutamide can prolong life in men with prostate cancer.
Echinococcosis	Echinococcosis, which is often times referred to as hydatid disease or echinococcal disease, is a parasitic disease that affects both humans and other mammals, such as sheep, dogs, rodents and horses. There are three different forms of echinococcosis found in humans, each of which is caused by the larval stages of different species of the tapeworm of genus Echinococcus. The first of the three and also the most common form found in humans is cystic echinococcosis which is caused by Echinococcus granulosus.
Echinococcus granulosus	Echinococcus granulosus, is a cyclophyllid cestode that parasitizes the small intestine of canids as an adult, but which has important intermediate hosts such as livestock and humans, where it causes hydatid disease. The adult tapeworm ranges in length from 2 mm to 7 mm and has three proglottids ("segments") when intact - an immature proglottid, mature proglottid and a gravid proglottid. Like all cyclophyllideans, E. granulosus has four suckers on its scolex ("head"), and E. granulosus also has a rostellum with hooks.

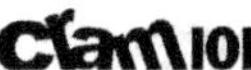

Gonorrhea	Gonorrhea is a common sexually transmitted infection caused by the bacterium Neisseria gonorrhoeae. The usual symptoms in men are burning with urination and penile discharge. Women, on the other hand, are asymptomatic half the time or have vaginal discharge and pelvic pain.
Herpes simplex	Herpes simplex is a viral disease caused by both herpes simplex virus type 1 (HSV-1) and type 2 (HSV-2). Infection with the herpes virus is categorized into one of several distinct disorders based on the site of infection. Oral herpes, the visible symptoms of which are colloquially called cold sores or fever blisters, infects the face and mouth.
Neisseria gonorrhoeae	Neisseria gonorrhoeae, or gonococcus, is a species of Gram-negative coffee bean-shaped diplococci bacteria responsible for the sexually transmitted infection gonorrhea. N. gonorrhoea was first described by Albert Neisser in 1879. Microbiology Neisseria are fastidious Gram-negative cocci that require nutrient supplementation to grow in laboratory cultures.
Trichomonas vaginalis	Trichomonas vaginalis is an anaerobic, flagellated protozoan, a form of microorganism. The parasitic microorganism is the causative agent of trichomoniasis, and is the most common pathogenic protozoan infection of humans in industrialized countries. Infection rates between men and women are the same with women showing symptoms while infections in men are usually asymptomatic.
Ureaplasma urealyticum	Ureaplasma urealyticum is a bacterium belonging to the family Mycoplasmataceae. Its type strain is T960. Clinical significance U. urealyticum is part of the normal genital flora of both men and women.

Urethritis	Urethritis is inflammation of the urethra. The main symptom is dysuria, which is painful or difficult urination. The disease is classified as either gonocococcal urethritis, caused by Neisseria gonorrhoeae, or non-gonococcal urethritis most commonly caused by Chlamydia trachomatis.
Erectile dysfunction	Erectile dysfunction is sexual dysfunction characterized by the inability to develop or maintain an erection of the penis during sexual performance. A penile erection is the hydraulic effect of blood entering and being retained in sponge-like bodies within the penis. The process is often initiated as a result of sexual arousal, when signals are transmitted from the brain to nerves in the penis.
Etiology	Etiology is the study of causation, or origination. The word is most commonly used in medical and philosophical theories, where it is used to refer to the study of why things occur, or even the reasons behind the way that things act, and is used in philosophy, physics, psychology, government, medicine, theology and biology in reference to the causes of various phenomena. An etiological myth is a myth intended to explain a name or create a mythic history for a place or family.
Infection	An infection is the colonization of a host organism by parasite species. Infecting parasites seek to use the host's resources to reproduce, often resulting in disease. Colloquially, infections are usually considered to be caused by microscopic organisms or microparasites like viruses, prions, bacteria, and viroids, though larger organisms like macroparasites and fungi can also infect.

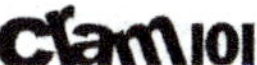

Chapter 2. PART II: Chapter 15 - Chapter 28

Infection	An infection is the colonization of a host organism by parasite species. Infecting parasites seek to use the host's resources to reproduce, often resulting in disease. Colloquially, infections are usually considered to be caused by microscopic organisms or microparasites like viruses, prions, bacteria, and viroids, though larger organisms like macroparasites and fungi can also infect.
Antiandrogen	An antiandrogen, is any of a group of hormone receptor antagonist compounds that are capable of preventing or inhibiting the biologic effects of androgens, male sex hormones, on normally responsive tissues in the body. Antiandrogens usually work by blocking the appropriate receptors, competing for binding sites on the cell's surface, obstructing the androgens' pathway. Indications Antiandrogens are often indicated to treat severe male sexual disorders, such as hypersexuality (excessive sexual desire) and sexual deviation such as paraphilias, as well as use as an antineoplastic agent and palliative, adjuvant or neoadjuvant hormonal therapy in prostate cancer.
Cephalosporin	The cephalosporins are a class of β-lactam antibiotics originally derived from Acremonium, which was previously known as "Cephalosporium". Together with cephamycins they constitute a subgroup of β-lactam antibiotics called cephems. History Cephalosporin compounds were first isolated from cultures of Cephalosporium acremonium from a sewer in Sardinia in 1948 by Italian scientist Giuseppe Brotzu.
Folliculitis	Folliculitis is the inflammation of one or more hair follicles. The condition may occur anywhere on the skin.

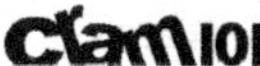

Most carbuncles, furuncles, and other cases of folliculitis develop from Staphylococcus aureus.

Genital ulcer

A Genital ulcer is an ulcer located on the genital area, usually caused by a sexually transmitted disease such as genital herpes, syphilis, chancroid, or thrush. Some other signs of having genital ulcers include enlarged lymph nodes in the groin area, or vesicular lesions, which are small, elevated sores or blisters. The syndrome may be further classified into penile ulceration and vulval ulceration for males and females respectively.

Laboratory

A laboratory is a facility that provides controlled conditions in which scientific research, experiments, and measurement may be performed. The title of laboratory is also used for certain other facilities where the processes or equipment used are similar to those in scientific laboratories. These notably include:

- the film laboratory or darkroom
- the computer lab
- the medical lab
- the public health lab
- the clandestine lab for the production of illegal drugs

In recent years government and private centers for innovation in learning, leadership and organization have adopted "lab" in their name to emphasize the experimental and research-oriented nature of their work.

Cervicitis

Cervicitis is inflammation of the uterine cervix. Cervicitis in women has many features in common with urethritis in men and many cases are caused by sexually transmitted infections. Non-infectious causes of cervicitis can include intrauterine devices, contraceptive diaphragms, and allergic reactions to spermicides or latex condoms.

Epididymitis

Epididymitis is a medical condition in which there is inflammation of the epididymis (a curved structure at the back of the testicle in which sperm matures and is stored). This condition may be mildly to very painful, and the scrotum (sac containing the testicles) may become red, warm and swollen. It may be acute (of sudden onset) or rarely chronic.

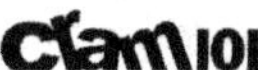

Herpes simplex virus	Herpes simplex virus 1 and 2 (Herpes simplex virus-1 and Herpes simplex virus-2), also known as Human herpes virus 1 and 2 (HHV-1 and -2), are two members of the herpes virus family, Herpesviridae, that infect humans. Both Herpes simplex virus-1 (which produces cold sores) and Herpes simplex virus-2 (which produces genital herpes) are ubiquitous and contagious. They can be spread when an infected person is producing and shedding the virus.
Syphilis	Syphilis is a sexually transmitted disease caused by the spirochetal bacteria Treponema pallidum subspecies pallidum. The primary route of transmission of syphilis is through sexual contact however it may also be transmitted from mother to fetus during pregnancy or at birth resulting in congenital syphilis. The signs and symptoms of syphilis vary depending on which of the four stages it presents in (primary, secondary, latent, and tertiary).
Chancroid	Chancroid is a sexually transmitted infection characterized by painful sores on the genitalia. Chancroid is known to be spread from one to another individual through sexual contact. Chancroid is a bacterial infection caused by the fastidious Gram-negative streptobacillus Haemophilus ducreyi.
Lymphogranuloma venereum	Lymphogranuloma venereum is a sexually transmitted disease caused by the invasive serovars L1, L2, L2a or L3 of Chlamydia trachomatis. LGV was first described by Wallace in 1833 and again by Durand, Nicolas, and Favre in 1913. Overview LGV is primarily an infection of lymphatics and lymph nodes.

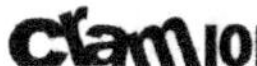

Penicillin	Penicillin is a group of antibiotics derived from Penicillium fungi. Penicillin antibiotics are historically significant because they are the first drugs that were effective against many previously serious diseases such as syphilis and Staphylococcus infections. Penicillins are still widely used today, though many types of bacteria are now resistant.
Pregnancy	Pregnancy is the carrying of one or more offspring, known as a fetus or embryo, inside the womb of a female. In a pregnancy, there can be multiple gestations, as in the case of twins or triplets. Human pregnancy is the most studied of all mammalian pregnancies.
Aminoglycoside	An aminoglycoside is a molecule or a portion of a molecule composed of amino-modified sugars. Several aminoglycosides function as antibiotics that are effective against certain types of bacteria. They include amikacin, arbekacin, gentamicin, kanamycin, neomycin, netilmicin, paromomycin, rhodostreptomycin, streptomycin, tobramycin, and apramycin.
Azathioprine	Azathioprine is a drug that suppresses the immune system. Azathioprine is used in organ transplantation and autoimmune disease. Some of the autoimmune diseases are rheumatoid arthritis, pemphigus, Inflammatory Bowel Disease (such as Crohn's disease and Ulcerative Colitis), multiple sclerosis, autoimmune hepatitis, atopic dermatitis, Myasthenia Gravis, Neuromyelitis Optica and restrictive lung disease.
Granuloma	Granuloma is a medical term for a roughly spherical mass of immune cells that forms when the immune system attempts to wall off substances that it perceives as foreign but is unable to eliminate. Such substances include infectious organisms such as bacteria and fungi as well as other materials such as keratin and suture fragments. A granuloma is therefore a special type of inflammation that can occur in a wide variety of diseases.

Granuloma inguinale	Granuloma inguinale is a bacterial disease characterized by ulcerative genital lesions that is endemic in many less developed regions. It is also known as donovanosis, granuloma genitoinguinale, granuloma inguinale tropicum, granuloma venereum, granuloma venereum genitoinguinale, lupoid form of groin ulceration, serpiginous ulceration of the groin, ulcerating granuloma of the pudendum and ulcerating sclerosing granuloma. The disease often goes untreated because of the scarcity of medical treatment in the countries in which it is found.
Human papillomavirus	Human papillomavirus is a member of the papillomavirus family of viruses that is capable of infecting humans. Like all papillomaviruses, HPVs establish productive infections only in the stratified epithelium of the skin or mucous membranes. While the majority of the nearly 200 known types of HPV cause no symptoms in most people, some types can cause warts (verrucae), while others can - in a minority of cases - lead to cancers of the cervix, vulva, vagina, and anus in women or cancers of the anus and penis in men.
Cancer	Cancer (medical term: malignant neoplasm) is a class of diseases in which a group of cells display uncontrolled growth, invasion that intrudes upon and destroys adjacent tissues, and sometimes metastasis, or spreading to other locations in the body via lymph or blood. These three malignant properties of cancers differentiate them from benign tumors, which do not invade or metastasize. Researchers divide the causes of cancer into two groups: those with an environmental cause and those with a hereditary genetic cause.
Genital wart	Genital warts (or Condylomata acuminata, venereal warts, anal warts and anogenital warts) is a highly contagious sexually transmitted disease caused by some sub-types of human papillomavirus (HPV). It is spread through direct skin-to-skin contact during oral, genital, or anal sex with an infected partner. Warts are the most easily recognized symptom of genital HPV infection, where types 6 and 11 are responsible for 90% of genital warts cases.
Prostate	The prostate is a compound tubuloalveolar exocrine gland of the male reproductive system in most mammals. In 2002, female paraurethral glands, or Skene's glands, were officially renamed the female prostate by the Federative International Committee on Anatomical Terminology.

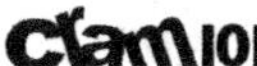

The prostate differs considerably among species anatomically, chemically, and physiologically.

Prostate cancer

Prostate cancer is a form of cancer that develops in the prostate, a gland in the male reproductive system. Most prostate cancers are slow growing; however, there are cases of aggressive prostate cancers. The cancer cells may metastasize (spread) from the prostate to other parts of the body, particularly the bones and lymph nodes.

Renal failure

Renal failure or kidney failure (formerly called renal insufficiency) describes a medical condition in which the kidneys fail to adequately filter toxins and waste products from the blood. The two forms are acute (acute kidney injury) and chronic (chronic kidney disease); a number of other diseases or health problems may cause either form of renal failure to occur.

Renal failure is described as a decrease in the glomerular filtration rate.

Urine

Urine is a sterile (in the absence of a disease condition), liquid by-product of the body that is secreted by the kidneys through a process called urination and excreted through the urethra. Cellular metabolism generates numerous by-products, many rich in nitrogen, that require elimination from the bloodstream. These by-products are eventually expelled from the body in a process known as micturition, the primary method for excreting water-soluble chemicals from the body.

Wart

A wart is generally a small, rough growth, typically on hands and feet but often other locations, that can resemble a cauliflower or a solid blister. They are caused by a viral infection, specifically by human papillomavirus 2 and 7. There are as many as 10 varieties of warts with the most common being considered largely harmless. It is possible to get warts from others; they are contagious.

Trauma

Trauma refers to "a body wound or shock produced by sudden physical injury, as from violence or accident." It can also be described as "a physical wound or injury, such as a fracture or blow." Major trauma can result in secondary complications such as circulatory shock, respiratory failure and death. Resuscitation of a trauma patient often involves multiple management procedures. Trauma is the sixth leading cause of death worldwide, accounting for 10% of all mortality, and is a serious public health problem with significant social and economic costs.

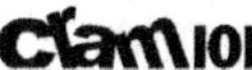

Oxalate	Oxalate is the dianion with formula $C_2O_4^{2-}$ also written $(COO)_2^{2-}$. Either name is often used for derivatives, such as disodium oxalate, $(Na^+)_2C_2O_4^{2-}$, or an ester of oxalic acid (such as dimethyl oxalate, $(CH_3)_2C_2O_4$. Oxalate also forms coordination compounds where it is sometimes abbreviated as ox.
Phosphate	A phosphate, an inorganic chemical, is a salt of phosphoric acid. In organic chemistry, a phosphate, or organophosphate, is an ester of phosphoric acid. Organic phosphates are important in biochemistry and biogeochemistry or ecology.
Sodium	Sodium is a metallic element with a symbol Na and atomic number 11. It is a soft, silvery-white, highly reactive metal and is a member of the alkali metals within "group 1" (formerly known as 'group IA'). It has only one stable isotope, ^{23}Na. Elemental sodium was first isolated by Humphry Davy in 1807 by passing an electric current through molten sodium hydroxide.
Uric acid	Uric acid is a heterocyclic compound of carbon, nitrogen, oxygen, and hydrogen with the formula $C_5H_4N_4O_3$. Uric acid is created when the body breaks down purine nucleotides. Chemistry Uric acid is a diprotic acid with pKa_1=5.4 and pKa_2=10.3. Thus in strong alkali at high pH, it forms the dually charged full urate ion, but at biological pH or in the presence of carbonic acid or carbonate ions, it forms the singly charged hydrogen or acid urate ion as its pKa_2 is greater than the pKa_1 of carbonic acid.
Citrate	A citrate can refer either to the conjugate base of citric acid, $(C_3H_5O(COO)_3^{3-})$, or to the esters of citric acid. An example of the former, a salt is trisodium citrate; an ester is triethyl citrate. Other citric acid ions

Since citric acid is a multifunctional acid, intermediate ions exist, hydrogen citrate ion, $HC_6H_5O_7^{2-}$ and dihydrogen citrate ion, $H_2C_6H_5O_7^{-}$.

Magnesium

Magnesium is a chemical element with the symbol Mg, atomic number 12 and common oxidation number +2. It is an alkaline earth metal and the seventh most abundant element in the Earth's crust, where it constitutes about 2% by mass, and ninth in the known Universe as a whole. This preponderance of magnesium is related to the fact that it is easily built up in supernova stars from a sequential addition of three helium nuclei to carbon (which in turn is made from three helium nuclei). Due to magnesium ion's high solubility in water, it is the third most abundant element dissolved in seawater.

Sulfate

In inorganic chemistry, a sulfate is a salt of sulfuric acid.

Chemical properties

The sulfate ion is a polyatomic anion with the empirical formula SO_{2-}

4 and a molecular mass of 96.06 daltons (96.06 g/mol); it consists of a central sulfur atom surrounded by four equivalent oxygen atoms in a tetrahedral arrangement. The symmetry is very similar to that of methane, CH_4.

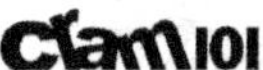

Cystitis	Cystitis is a term that refers to urinary bladder inflammation that results from any one of a number of distinct syndromes . It is most commonly caused by a bacterial infection in which case it is referred to as a urinary tract infection. Signs and symptoms • Pressure in the lower pelvis • Painful urination (dysuria) • Frequent urination (polyuria) or urgent need to urinate (urinary urgency) • Need to urinate at night (nocturia, similar to prostate cancer or BPH) • Abnormal urine color (cloudy), similar to a urinary tract infection • Foul or strong urine odor Differential diagnosis There are several medically distinct types of cystitis, each having a unique etiology and therapeutic approach: • Traumatic cystitis is probably the most common form of cystitis in the female, and is due to bruising of the bladder, usually by abnormally forceful sexual intercourse.
Hyperoxaluria	Hyperoxaluria is an excessive urinary excretion of oxalate. Individuals with hyperoxaluria often have calcium oxalate kidney stones. Type I (PH1) is associated with AGXT protein, a key enzyme involved in breakdown of oxalate.
Stress incontinence	Stress incontinence is a form of urinary incontinence. Stress urinary incontinence (SUI), also known as effort incontinence, is due essentially to insufficient strength of the pelvic floor muscles. Pathophysiology

It is the loss of small amounts of urine associated with coughing, laughing, sneezing, exercising or other movements that increase intra-abdominal pressure and thus increase pressure on the bladder.

Struvite

Struvite is a phosphate mineral with formula: $NH_4MgPO_4 \cdot 6H_2O$. Struvite crystallizes in the orthorhombic system as white to yellowish or brownish-white pyramidal crystals or in platey mica-like forms. It is a soft mineral with Mohs hardness of 1.5 to 2 and has a low specific gravity of 1.7. It is sparingly soluble in neutral and alkaline conditions, but readily soluble in acid.

Struvite urinary stones and crystals form readily in the urine of animals and humans that are infected with ammonia-producing organisms.

Cystine

Cystine is a dimeric amino acid formed by the oxidation of two cysteine residues that covalently link to make a disulfide bond. This organosulfur compound has the formula $(SCH_2CH(NH_2)CO_2H)_2$. It is a white solid, and melts at 247-249 °C. It was discovered in 1810 by William Hyde Wollaston but was not recognized as being derived of proteins until it was isolated from the horn of a cow in 1899. Through formation of disulfide bonds within and between protein molecules, cystine is a significant determinant of the tertiary structure of most proteins.

Filariasis

Filariasis is a parasitic disease and is considered an infectious tropical disease, that is caused by thread-like filarial nematodes (roundworms) in the superfamily Filarioidea, also known as "filariae".

In humans

There are 8 known filarial nematodes which use humans as the host. These are divided into 3 groups according to the niche within the body that they occupy: 'lymphatic filariasis', 'subcutaneous filariasis', and 'serous cavity filariasis'.

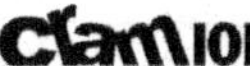

Xanthine	Xanthine, (3,7-dihydro-purine-2,6-dione), is a purine base found in most human body tissues and fluids and in other organisms. A number of mild stimulants are derived from xanthine, including caffeine and theobromine. Xanthine is a product on the pathway of purine degradation.
Silicate	A silicate is a compound containing a silicon bearing anion.
Indinavir	Indinavir is a protease inhibitor used as a component of highly active antiretroviral therapy (HAART) to treat HIV infection and AIDS. History The Food and Drug Administration (FDA) approved indinavir March 13, 1996, making it the eighth approved antiretroviral. Indinavir was much more powerful than any prior antiretroviral drug; using it with dual NRTIs set the standard for treatment of HIV/AIDS and raised the bar on design and introduction of subsequent antiretroviral drugs. Protease inhibitors changed the very nature of the AIDS epidemic from one of a terminal illness to a somewhat manageable one.
Pain	Pain is "an unpleasant sensory and emotional experience associated with actual or potential tissue damage, or described in terms of such damage." It is the feeling common to such experiences as stubbing a toe, burning a finger, putting iodine on a cut, and bumping the "funny bone". Pain motivates us to withdraw from potentially damaging situations, protect a damaged body part while it heals, and avoid those situations in the future. Most pain resolves promptly once the painful stimulus is removed and the body has healed, but sometimes pain persists despite removal of the stimulus and apparent healing of the body; and sometimes pain arises in the absence of any detectable stimulus, damage or disease.

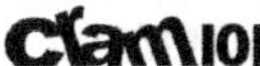

Triamterene	Triamterene is a potassium-sparing diuretic used in combination with thiazide diuretics for the treatment of hypertension and edema. Mechanism of action Triamterene directly blocks the epithelial sodium channel (ENaC) on the lumen side of the kidney collecting tubule. Other diuretics cause a decrease in the sodium concentration of the forming urine due to the entry of sodium into the cell via the ENaC, and the concomitant exit of potassium from the principal cell into the forming urine.
Hematuria	In medicine, hematuria, is the presence of red blood cells (erythrocytes) in the urine. It may be idiopathic and/or benign, or it can be a sign that there is a kidney stone or a tumor in the urinary tract (kidneys, ureters, urinary bladder, prostate, and urethra), ranging from trivial to lethal. If white blood cells are found in addition to red blood cells, then it is a signal of urinary tract infection.
Urinary incontinence	Urinary incontinence is any involuntary leakage of urine. It is a common and distressing problem, which may have a profound impact on quality of life. Urinary incontinence almost always results from an underlying treatable medical condition but is under-reported to medical practitioners.
Schistosomiasis	Schistosomiasis is a parasitic disease caused by several species of trematodes (platyhelminth infection, or "flukes"), a parasitic worm of the genus Schistosoma. Although it has a low mortality rate, schistosomiasis often is a chronic illness that can damage internal organs and, in children, impair growth and cognitive development. The urinary form of schistosomiasis is associated with increased risks for bladder cancer in adults.
Pyonephrosis	Pyonephrosis is an infection of the renal collecting system. Pus collects in the renal pelvis and causes distension of the kidney.

	It can cause kidney failure.
Kidney	The kidneys are organs with several functions. They are seen in many types of animals, including vertebrates and some invertebrates. They are an essential part of the urinary system and also serve homeostatic functions such as the regulation of electrolytes, maintenance of acid-base balance, and regulation of blood pressure.
Nephrectomy	Nephrectomy is the surgical removal of a kidney. History The first successful nephrectomy was performed by the German surgeon Gustav Simon on August 2, 1869 in Heidelberg. Simon practiced the operation beforehand in animal experiments.
Symptom	A symptom is a departure from normal function or feeling which is noticed by a patient, indicating the presence of disease or abnormality. A symptom is subjective, observed by the patient, and not measured. A symptom may not be a malady, for example symptoms of pregnancy.
Voiding cystourethrogram	In urology, a voiding cystourethrogram also micturating cystourethrogram (MCUG), is a technique for watching a person's urethra and urinary bladder while the person urinates (voids). The technique consists of catheterizing the person in order to fill the bladder with a radiopaque liquid (a "contrast" or "contrast agent", typically cystografin). Under fluoroscopy (real time x-rays) the radiologist watches the contrast enter the bladder and looks at the anatomy of the patient.
Medullary sponge kidney	Also known as Cacchi Ricci disease, medullary sponge kidney is a congenital disorder of the kidneys characterized by cystic dilatation of the collecting tubules in one or both kidneys. It has been estimated to occur with a frequency of 1 in every 5,000 individuals in a population. The disease is bilateral in 70% of cases.

Renal tubular acidosis	Renal tubular acidosis is a medical condition that involves an accumulation of acid in the body due to a failure of the kidneys to appropriately acidify the urine. When blood is filtered by the kidney, the filtrate passes through the tubules of the nephron, allowing for exchange of salts, acid equivalents, and other solutes before it drains into the bladder as urine. The metabolic acidosis that results from Renal tubular acidosis may be caused either by failure to recover sufficient (alkaline) bicarbonate ions from the filtrate in the early portion of the nephron (proximal tubule) or by insufficient secretion of (acid) hydrogen ions into the latter portions of the nephron (distal tubule).
Tumor	A tumor is the name for a neoplasm or a solid lesion formed by an abnormal growth of cells (termed neoplastic) which looks like a swelling. Tumor is not synonymous with cancer. A tumor can be benign, pre-malignant or malignant, whereas cancer is by definition malignant.
Crystalluria	Crystalluria refers to crystals found in the urine when performing a urine test. Clinical significance It can be an indication of urolithiasis. It can be associated with cysteinuria.
Diagnosis	Diagnosis is the identification of the nature and cause of anything. Diagnosis is used in many different disciplines with variations in the use of logics, analytics, and experience to determine the cause and effect relationships. In systems engineering and computer science, diagnosis is typically used to determine the causes of symptoms, mitigations for problems, and solutions to issues.
Differential diagnosis	A differential diagnosis is a systematic method used to identify unknowns. This method, essentially a process of elimination, is used by taxonomists to identify living organisms, and by physicians, nurse practitioners, physician assistants, and other trained medical professionals to diagnose the specific disease in a patient.

	Not all medical diagnoses are differential ones: some diagnoses merely name a set of signs and symptoms that may have more than one possible cause, and some diagnoses are based on intuition or estimations of likelihood.
Risk factor	In epidemiology, a risk factor is a variable associated with an increased risk of disease or infection. Sometimes, determinant is also used, being a variable associated with either increased or decreased risk. Risk factors or determinants are correlational and not necessarily causal, because correlation does not imply causation.
Physical examination	Physical examination is the process by which a doctor investigates the body of a patient for signs of disease. It generally follows the taking of the medical history -- an account of the symptoms as experienced by the patient. Together with the medical history, the physical examination aids in determining the correct diagnosis and devising the treatment plan.
Intravenous pyelogram	An intravenous pyelogram is a radiological procedure used to visualize abnormalities of the urinary system, including the kidneys, ureters, and bladder. Procedure An injection of x-ray contrast media is given to a patient via a needle or cannula into the vein, typically in the arm. The contrast is excreted or removed from the bloodstream via the kidneys, and the contrast media becomes visible on x-rays almost immediately after injection.
Pyelogram	Pyelogram is a form of imaging of the renal pelvis and ureter. Types include: • Intravenous pyelogram • Retrograde pyelogram .

Tomography	Tomography is imaging by sections or sectioning, through the use of any kind of penetrating wave. A device used in tomography is called a tomograph, while the image produced is a tomogram. The method is used in radiology, archaeology, biology, geophysics, oceanography, materials science, astrophysics and other sciences.
Extracorporeal shock wave lithotripsy	Extracorporeal shock wave lithotripsy is the non-invasive treatment of kidney stones (urinary calculosis) and biliary calculi (stones in the gallbladder or in the liver) using an acoustic pulse. Lithotripsy and the lithotriptor were developed in the early 1980s in Germany by Dornier Medizintechnik GmbH (now known as Dornier MedTech Systems GmbH), and came into widespread use with the introduction of the HM-3 lithotriptor in 1983. Within a few years, Extracorporeal shock wave lithotripsy became a standard treatment of calculosis. It is estimated that more than one million patients are treated annually with Extracorporeal shock wave lithotripsy in the USA alone.
Percutaneous	In surgery, percutaneous pertains to any medical procedure where access to inner organs or other tissue is done via needle-puncture of the skin, rather than by using an "open" approach where inner organs or tissue are exposed (typically with the use of a scalpel). The percutaneous approach is commonly used in vascular procedures. This involves a needle catheter getting access to a blood vessel, followed by the introduction of a wire through the lumen (pathway) of the needle.
Percutaneous nephrolithotomy	Percutaneous nephrolithotomy is a surgical procedure to remove stones from the kidney by a small puncture wound (up to about 1 cm) through the skin. It is most suitable to remove stones of more than 2 cm in size. It is usually done under general anesthesia or spinal anesthesia.
Nephrotomy	Nephrotomy describes a surgical procedure in which the kidney is cut.
Seminal vesicle	The seminal vesicles (glandulae vesiculosae) or vesicular glands are a pair of simple tubular glands posteroinferior to the urinary bladder of male mammals. Anatomy

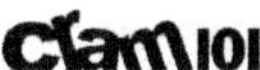

Each seminal gland spreads approximately 5 cm, though the full length of seminal vesicle is approximately 10 cm, but it is curled up inside of the gland's structure. Each gland forms as an outpocketing of the wall of ampulla of each vas deferens.

Anatomy

Anatomy is a branch of biology and medicine that is the consideration of the structure of living things. It is a general term that includes human anatomy, animal anatomy and plant anatomy. In some of its facets anatomy is closely related to embryology, comparative anatomy and comparative embryology, through common roots in evolution.

Histology

Histology is the study of the microscopic anatomy of cells and tissues of plants and animals. It is performed by examining a thin slice (section) of tissue under a light microscope or electron microscope. The ability to visualize or differentially identify microscopic structures is frequently enhanced through the use of histological stains.

Renal pelvis

The renal pelvis is the funnel-like dilated proximal part of the ureter in the kidney.

In humans, the renal pelvis is the point of convergence of two or three major calyces. Each renal papilla is surrounded by a branch of the renal pelvis called a calyx.

Ureter

In human anatomy, the ureters are muscular tubes that propel urine from the kidneys to the urinary bladder. In the adult, the ureters are usually 25-30 cm (10-12 in) long and ~3-4 mm in diameter.

In humans, the ureters arise from the renal pelvis on the medial aspect of each kidney before descending towards the bladder on the front of the psoas major muscle.

Actinomycosis

Actinomycosis is an infectious bacterial disease caused by Actinomyces species such as Actinomyces israelii or A. gerencseriae. It can also be caused by Propionibacterium propionicus, and the condition is likely to be polymicrobial.

	Actinomycosis occurs rarely in humans but rather frequently in cattle as a disease called lumpy jaw.
Pathology	Pathology is the study and diagnosis of disease. The word pathology is from Greek π?θος, pathos, "feeling, suffering"; and -λογ?α, -logia, "the study of". Pathologization, to pathologize, refers to the process of defining a condition or behavior as pathological, e.g. pathological gambling.
Tuberculosis	Tuberculosis, MTB or TB (short for tubercles bacillus) is a common and in some cases deadly infectious disease caused by various strains of mycobacteria, usually Mycobacterium tuberculosis in humans. Tuberculosis usually attacks the lungs but can also affect other parts of the body. It is spread through the air when people who have active MTB infection cough, sneeze, or spit.
Hydronephrosis	Hydronephrosis is distension and dilation of the renal pelvis calyces, usually caused by obstruction of the free flow of urine from the kidney, leading to progressive atrophy of the kidney. In cases of hydroureteronephrosis, there is distention of both the ureter and the renal pelvis and calices. Signs and symptoms The signs and symptoms of hydronephrosis depend upon whether the obstruction is acute or chronic, partial or complete, unilateral or bilateral.
Pathogenesis	The term pathogenesis means step by step development of a disease and the chain of events leading to that disease due to a series of changes in the structure and/or function of a cell/tissue/organ being caused by a microbial, chemical or physical agent. The pathogenesis of a disease is the mechanism by which a disease is caused. The term can also be used to describe the development of the disease, such as acute, chronic and recurrent.

Vascular	Vascular in zoology and medicine means "related to blood vessels", which are part of the circulatory system. An organ or tissue that is vascularized is heavily endowed with blood vessels and thus richly supplied with blood. In botany, plants with a dedicated transport system for water and nutrients are called vascular plants.
Prognosis	Prognosis is a medical term to describe the likely outcome of an illness. When applied to large populations, prognostic estimates can be very accurate: for example the statement "45% of patients with severe septic shock will die within 28 days" can be made with some confidence, because previous research found that this proportion of patients died. However, it is much harder to translate this into a prognosis for an individual patient: additional information is needed to determine whether a patient belongs to the 45% who will succumb, or to the 55% who survive.
Scrotum	In some male mammals the scrotum is a dual-chambered protuberance of skin and muscle containing the testicles and divided by a septum. It is an extension of the abdomen, and is located between the penis and anus. In humans and some other mammals, the base of the scrotum becomes covered with curly pubic hairs at puberty.
Sertoli cell	A Sertoli cell is a 'nurse' cell of the testes that is part of a seminiferous tubule. It is activated by follicle-stimulating hormone and has FSH-receptor on its membranes. Functions Because its main function is to nurture the developing sperm cells through the stages of spermatogenesis, the Sertoli cell has also been called the "mother" or "nurse" cell.

Antigen	An antigen is a substance/molecule that, when introduced into the body, triggers the production of an antibody by the immune system, which will then kill or neutralize the antigen that is recognized as a foreign and potentially harmful invader. These invaders can be molecules such as pollen or cells such as bacteria. The term originally came from antibody generator and was a molecule that binds specifically to an antibody, but the term now also refers to any molecule or molecular fragment that can be bound by a major histocompatibility complex (MHC) and presented to a T-cell receptor.
Germ cell	A germ cell is any biological cell that gives rise to the gametes of an organism that reproduces sexually. In many animals, the germ cells originate near the gut of an embryo and migrate to the developing gonads. There, they undergo cell division of two types, mitosis and meiosis, followed by cellular differentiation into mature gametes, either eggs or sperm.
Immunotherapy	Immunotherapy is a medical term defined as "treatment of disease by inducing, enhancing, or suppressing an immune response". Immunotherapies designed to elicit or amplify an immune response are classified as activation immunotherapies. Immunotherapies designed to reduce, suppress or more appropriately direct an existing immune response, as in cases of autoimmunity or allergy, are classified as suppression immunotherapies.
Monoclonal antibodies	Monoclonal antibodies are monospecific antibodies that are the same because they are made by identical immune cells that are all clones of a unique parent cell. Given almost any substance, it is possible to produce monoclonal antibodies that specifically bind to that substance; they can then serve to detect or purify that substance. This has become an important tool in biochemistry, molecular biology and medicine.
Radioimmunodetection	Radioimmunodetection is an imaging technique using radiolabeled antibodies.

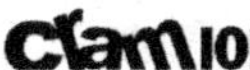

Chapter 2. PART II: Chapter 15 - Chapter 28

Cancer	Cancer (medical term: malignant neoplasm) is a class of diseases in which a group of cells display uncontrolled growth, invasion that intrudes upon and destroys adjacent tissues, and sometimes metastasis, or spreading to other locations in the body via lymph or blood. These three malignant properties of cancers differentiate them from benign tumors, which do not invade or metastasize. Researchers divide the causes of cancer into two groups: those with an environmental cause and those with a hereditary genetic cause.
Cell-mediated immunity	Cell-mediated immunity is an immune response that does not involve antibodies or complement but rather involves the activation of macrophages, natural killer cells (NK), antigen-specific cytotoxic T-lymphocytes, and the release of various cytokines in response to an antigen. Historically, the immune system was separated into two branches: humoral immunity, for which the protective function of immunization could be found in the humor (cell-free bodily fluid or serum) and cellular immunity, for which the protective function of immunization was associated with cells. CD4 cells or helper T cells provide protection against different pathogens.
Infertility	Infertility primarily refers to the biological inability of a person to contribute to conception. Infertility may also refer to the state of a woman who is unable to carry a pregnancy to full term. There are many biological causes of infertility, some which may be bypassed with medical intervention.
Prostate-specific antigen	Prostate-specific antigen is a protein produced by the cells of the prostate gland. Prostate specific antigen is present in small quantities in the serum of men with healthy prostates, but is often elevated in the presence of prostate cancer and in other prostate disorders. A blood test to measure Prostate specific antigen is considered the most effective test currently available for the early detection of prostate cancer, but this effectiveness has also been questioned.
Vaccination	Vaccination is the administration of antigenic material (a vaccine) to stimulate adaptive immunity to a disease. Vaccines can prevent or ameliorate the effects of infection by many pathogens. There is strong evidence for the efficacy of many vaccines, such as the influenza vaccine, the HPV vaccine and the chicken pox vaccine among others.
Bladder cancer	Bladder cancer refers to any of several types of malignant growths of the urinary bladder. It is a disease in which abnormal cells multiply without control in the bladder. The bladder is a hollow, muscular organ that stores urine; it is located in the pelvis.

Carcinoma	Carcinoma is the medical condition of an invasive malignant tumor consisting of transformed epithelial cells. Alternatively, it refers to a malignant tumor composed of transformed cells of unknown histogenesis, but which possess specific molecular or histological characteristics that are associated with epithelial cells, such as the production of cytokeratins or intercellular bridges.
Renal cell carcinoma	Renal cell carcinoma is a kidney cancer that originates in the lining of the proximal convoluted tubule, the very small tubes in the kidney that filter the blood and remove waste products. Renal cell carcinoma is the most common type of kidney cancer in adults, responsible for approximately 80% of cases. It is also known to be the most lethal of all the genitourinary tumors.
Chemotherapy	Chemotherapy, in the most simple sense, is the treatment of an ailment by chemicals especially by killing micro-organisms or cancerous cells. In popular usage, it refers to antineoplastic drugs used to treat cancer or the combination of these drugs into a cytotoxic standardized treatment regimen. In its non-oncological use, the term may also refer to antibiotics (antibacterial chemotherapy).
Toxicity	Toxicity is the degree to which a substance can damage an organism. Toxicity can refer to the effect on a whole organism, such as an animal, bacterium, or plant, as well as the effect on a substructure of the organism, such as a cell (cytotoxicity) or an organ (organotoxicity), such as the liver (hepatotoxicity). By extension, the word may be metaphorically used to describe toxic effects on larger and more complex groups, such as the family unit or society at large.
Renal function	Renal function, in nephrology, is an indication of the state of the kidney and its role in renal physiology. Glomerular filtration rate (GFR) describes the flow rate of filtered fluid through the kidney. Creatinine clearance rate (C_{Cr} or CrCl) is the volume of blood plasma that is cleared of creatinine per unit time and is a useful measure for approximating the GFR. Creatinine clearance exceeds GFR due to creatinine secretion, which can be blocked by cimetidine.
Surgery	Surgery is an ancient medical specialty that uses operative manual and instrumental techniques on a patient to investigate and/or treat a pathological condition such as disease or injury, to help improve bodily function or appearance, and sometimes for religious reasons. An act of performing surgery may be called a surgical procedure, operation, or simply surgery. In this context, the verb operate means performing surgery.

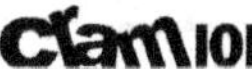

Transitional cell carcinoma	Transitional cell carcinoma is a type of cancer that typically occurs in the urinary system: the kidney, urinary bladder, and accessory organs. It is the most common type of bladder cancer and cancer of the ureter, urethra, and urachus; it is the second most common type of kidney cancer. Transitional cell carcinoma arises from the transitional epithelium, a tissue lining the inner surface of these hollow organs.
Histopathology	Histopathology refers to the microscopic examination of tissue in order to study the manifestations of disease. Specifically, in clinical medicine, histopathology refers to the examination of a biopsy or surgical specimen by a pathologist, after the specimen has been processed and histological sections have been placed onto glass slides. In contrast, cytopathology examines free cells or tissue fragments.
Cystectomy	Cystectomy is a medical term for surgical removal of all or part of the urinary bladder. It may also be rarely used to refer to the removal of a cyst, or the gallbladder. The most common condition warranting removal of the urinary bladder is bladder cancer.
Angiomyolipoma	Angiomyolipoma are the most common benign tumour of the kidney and are composed of blood vessels, smooth muscle cells and fat cells. Angiomyolipoma are strongly associated with the genetic disease tuberous sclerosis, in which most individuals will have several angiomyolipoma affecting both kidneys. They are also commonly found in women with the rare lung disease lymphangioleiomyomatosis.
Folliculin	Folliculin, BHD, FLCL, FLCN_HUMAN, MGC17998, or MGC23445 is a tumor-suppressor protein associated with Birt-Hogg-Dubé syndrome. It is encoded by the Folliculin gene sometimes also referred to as the BHD gene. The function of the folliculin protein has yet to be determined but current research suggests it may act as a tumor suppressor.

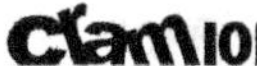

Oncocytoma	An oncocytoma is a tumor made up of oncocytes, a special kind of cells. Presentation An oncocytoma is an epithelial tumor composed of oncocytes, large eosinophilic cells having small, round, benign-appearing nuclei with large nucleoli. Oncocytoma can arise in a number of organs.
Adenocarcinoma	Adenocarcinoma is a cancer of an epithelium that originates in glandular tissue. Epithelial tissue includes, but is not limited to, the surface layer of skin, glands and a variety of other tissue that lines the cavities and organs of the body. Epithelium can be derived embryologically from ectoderm, endoderm or mesoderm.
Lymphangioleiomyomatosis	Lymphangioleiomyomatosis is a rare lung disease that results in a proliferation of disorderly smooth muscle growth (leiomyoma) throughout the bronchioles, alveolar septa, perivascular spaces, and lymphatics, resulting in the obstruction of small airways (leading to pulmonary cy formation and pneumothorax) and lymphatics (leading to chylous pleural effusion). LAM occu a sporadic form, which only affects females, who are usually of childbearing age. LAM also o in patients who have tuberous sclerosis.

Leiomyoma	A leiomyoma is a benign smooth muscle neoplasm that is not premalignant. They can occur in any organ, but the most common forms occur in the uterus, small bowel and the esophagus.
	
	Etymology
	
	• Greek:
	    ○ λε?ος leios "smooth"
	    ○ μ?ς mus (cf.

Lipoma	A lipoma is a benign tumor composed of adipose tissue. It is the most common form of soft tissue tumor. Lipomas are soft to the touch, usually movable, and are generally painless.

Epididymis	The epididymis is part of the male reproductive system and is present in all male amniotes. It is a narrow, tightly-coiled tube connecting the efferent ducts from the rear of each testicle to its vas deferens. A similar, but probably non-homologous, structure is found in cartilaginous fishes.
Juxtaglomerular cell tumor	Juxtaglomerular cell tumor is a rare kidney cancer that typically secretes renin. It involves the juxtaglomerular cells. It often causes hypertension, in adults and children, although among causes of hypertension it is rare.
Reflux	Reflux is a technique involving the condensation of vapors and the return of this condensate to the system from which it originated. It is used in industrial and laboratory distillations. It is also used in chemistry to supply energy to reactions over a long period of time.
Vesicoureteral reflux	Vesicoureteral reflux is an abnormal movement of urine from the bladder into ureters or kidneys. Urine normally travels from the kidneys via the ureters to the bladder. In vesicoureteral reflux the direction of urine flow is reversed (retrograde).
Paraneoplastic syndrome	A paraneoplastic syndrome is a disease or symptom that is the consequence of the presence of cancer in the body, but is not due to the local presence of cancer cells. These phenomena are mediated by humoral factors (by hormones or cytokines) excreted by tumor cells or by an immune response against the tumor. Paraneoplastic syndromes are typical among middle aged to older patients, and they most commonly present with cancers of the lung, breast, ovaries or lymphatic system (a lymphoma).
Disseminated disease	Disseminated disease refers to a diffuse disease process, generally either infectious or neoplastic, but sometimes also referring to connective tissue disease. A disseminated infection, for example, is one that has extended beyond its origin or nidus and involved the bloodstream to "seed" other areas of the body. Similarly, metastatic cancer can be viewed as a disseminated infection in that it has extended into the bloodstream or the lymphatic system to "seed" distant sites (known as metastasis).
Sarcoma	A sarcoma is a cancer that arises from transformed connective tissue cells. These cells originate from embryonic mesoderm, or middle layer, which forms the bone, cartilage, and fat tissues.

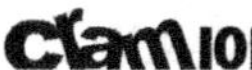

This is in contrast to carcinomas, which originate in the epithelium.

Benign prostatic hyperplasia

Benign prostatic hyperplasia also known as benign prostatic hypertrophy (technically a misnomer), benign enlargement of the prostate (BEP), and adenofibromyomatous hyperplasia, refers to the increase in size of the prostate.

To be accurate, the process is one of hyperplasia rather than hypertrophy, but the nomenclature is often interchangeable, even amongst urologists. It is characterized by hyperplasia of prostatic stromal and epithelial cells, resulting in the formation of large, fairly discrete nodules in the periurethral region of the prostate.

Epidemiology

Epidemiology is the study of patterns of health and illness and associated factors at the population level. It is the cornerstone method of public health research, and helps inform evidence-based medicine for identifying risk factors for disease and determining optimal treatment approaches to clinical practice and for preventative medicine. In the study of communicable and non-communicable diseases, epidemiologists are involved in outbreak investigation to study design, data collection, statistical analysis, documentation of results and submission for publication.

Pathophysiology

Pathophysiology is the study of the changes of normal mechanical, physical, and biochemical functions, either caused by a disease, or resulting from an abnormal syndrome. More formally, it is the branch of medicine which deals with any disturbances of body functions, caused by disease or prodromal symptoms.

An alternative definition is "the study of the biological and physical manifestations of disease as they correlate with the underlying abnormalities and physiological disturbances."

The study of pathology and the study of pathophysiology often involves substantial overlap in diseases and processes, but pathology emphasizes direct observations, while pathophysiology emphasizes quantifiable measurements.

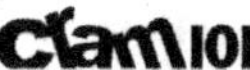

Cystoscopy	Cystoscopy is endoscopy of the urinary bladder via the urethra. It is carried out with a cystoscope. Diagnostic cystoscopy is usually carried out with local anaesthesia.
Watchful waiting	Watchful waiting is an approach to a medical problem in which time is allowed to pass before medical intervention or therapy is used. During this time, repeated testing may be performed. Related terms include expectant management, active surveillance and masterly inactivity.
Phytotherapy	Phytotherapy is the study of the use of extracts from natural origin as medicines or health-promoting agents. Traditional phytotherapy is often used as synonym for herbalism and regarded as "alternative medicine" by much of Western medicine. Modern phytotherapy when critically conducted, can be considered the scientific study on the effects and clinical use of herbal medicines.
Rectocele	A rectocele results from a tear in the rectovaginal septum (which is normally a tough, fibrous, sheet-like divider between the rectum and vagina). Rectal tissue bulges through this tear and into the vagina as a hernia. There are two main causes of this tear: childbirth, and hysterectomy.
Laser	A laser is a device that emits light (electromagnetic radiation) through a process of optical amplification based on the stimulated emission of photons. The term "laser" originated as an acronym for Light Amplification by Stimulated Emission of Radiation. The emitted laser light is notable for its high degree of spatial and temporal coherence, unattainable using other technologies.

Prostatectomy	A prostatectomy is the surgical removal of all or part of the prostate gland. Abnormalities of the prostate, such as a tumour, or if the gland itself becomes enlarged for any reason, can restrict the normal flow of urine along the urethra. There are several forms of the operation: Transurethral resection of the prostate (TURP) A cystoscope [a resectoscope which has a 30 degree viewing angle, along with resectoscopy sheath ' working element] is passed up the urethra to the prostate, where the surrounding prostate tissue is excised.
Laser surgery	Laser surgery is surgery using a laser to cut tissue instead of a scalpel. Examples include the use of a laser scalpel in otherwise conventional surgery, and soft tissue laser surgery, in which the laser beam vaporizes soft tissue with high water content. Laser resurfacing is a technique in which molecular bonds of a material are dissolved by a laser.
Transurethral incision of the prostate	Transurethral incision of the prostate is a surgical procedure for treating prostate gland enlargement (benign prostatic hyperplasia). Benefits Transurethral incision of the prostate---one or two small cuts in the prostate gland--can improve urine flow and correct other problems related to an enlarged prostate. Indications Compared with other surgical procedures for prostate gland enlargement, TUIP is simpler and generally has fewer complications.

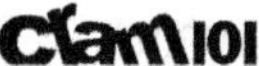

Transurethral resection of the prostate	Transurethral resection of the prostate is a urological operation. It is used to treat benign prostatic hyperplasia (BPH). As the name indicates, it is performed by visualising the prostate through the urethra and removing tissue by electrocautery or sharp dissection.
Hyperthermia	Hyperthermia is an elevated body temperature due to failed thermoregulation. Hyperthermia occurs when the body produces or absorbs more heat than it can dissipate. When the elevated body temperatures are sufficiently high, hyperthermia is a medical emergency and requires immediate treatment to prevent disability or death.
Transurethral needle ablation	Transurethral needle ablation is a procedure that is used to treat benign prostatic hypertrophy (BPH). A small probe that gives off low-level radiofrequency energy is inserted through the urethra into the prostate. The energy from the probe heats and destroys the abnormal prostate tissue without damaging the urethra.
Molecular genetics	Molecular genetics is the field of biology and genetics that studies the structure and function of genes at a molecular level. The field studies how the genes are transferred from generation to generation. Molecular genetics employs the methods of genetics and molecular biology.
Density	The mass density is defined as its mass per unit volume. The symbol most often used for density is ρ . In some cases (for instance, in the United States oil and gas industry), density is also defined as its weight per unit volume; although, this quantity is more properly called specific weight.
Detection	In general, detection is the extraction of particular information from a larger stream of information without specific cooperation from or synchronization with the sender. In the history of radio communications, the term "detector" was first used for a device that detected the simple presence or absence of a radio signal, since all communications were in Morse code. The term is still in use today to describe a component that extracts a particular signal from all of the electromagnetic waves present.
Reference range	In health-related fields, a reference range or reference interval usually describes the variations of a measurement or value in healthy individuals. It is a basis for a physician or other health professional to interpret a set of results for a particular patient.

The standard definition of a reference range basically originates in what is most prevalent in a control group taken from the population.

Tumor marker

A tumor marker is a substance found in the blood, urine, or body tissues that can be elevated in cancer, among other tissue types. There are many different tumor markers, each indicative of a particular disease process, and they are used in oncology to help detect the presence of cancer. An elevated level of a tumor marker can indicate cancer; however, there can also be other causes of the elevation.

Velocity

In physics, velocity is the measurement of the rate and direction of change in the position of an object. It is a vector physical quantity; both magnitude and direction are required to define it. The scalar absolute value (magnitude) of velocity is speed, a quantity that is measured in meters per second (m/s or ms^{-1}) when using the SI (metric) system.

Prostate biopsy

Prostate biopsy is a procedure in which small samples are removed from a man's prostate gland to be tested for the presence of cancer. It is typically performed when the scores from a PSA blood test rise to a level that is associated with the possible presence of prostate cancer.

The procedure, usually an outpatient procedure, requires a local anesthetic, with fifty-five percent of men reporting discomfort during the biopsy.

Quinolone

The quinolones are a family of synthetic broad-spectrum antibiotics. The term quinolone(s) refers to potent synthetic chemotherapeutic antibacterials.

The first generation of the quinolones begins with the introduction of nalidixic acid in 1962 for treatment of urinary tract infections in humans.

External beam radiotherapy

External beam radiotherapy otherwise known as teletherapy, is the most frequently used form of radiotherapy. The patient sits or lies on a couch and an external source of radiation is pointed at a particular part of the body. In contrast to internal radiotherapy (brachytherapy), in which the radiation source is placed inside the body, external beam radiotherapy directs the radiation at the tumour from outside the body.

Localized disease

A localized disease is an infectious or neoplastic process that originates in and is confined to one organ system or general area in the body, such as a sprained ankle, a boil on the hand, an abscess of finger.

A localized cancer that has not extended beyond the margins of the organ involved can also be described as localized disease, while cancers that extend into other tissues are described as invasive. Tumors that are non-hematologic in origin but extend into the bloodstream or lymphatic system are known as metastatic.

Brachytherapy

Brachytherapy, sealed source radiotherapy, curietherapy or endocurietherapy, is a form of radiotherapy where a radiation source is placed inside or next to the area requiring treatment. Brachytherapy is commonly used as an effective treatment for cervical, prostate, breast, and skin cancer and can also be used to treat tumours in many other body sites. Brachytherapy can be used alone or in combination with other therapies such as surgery, External Beam Radiotherapy (EBRT) and chemotherapy.

Androgen

Androgen, is the generic term for any natural or synthetic compound, usually a steroid hormone, that stimulates or controls the development and maintenance of male characteristics in vertebrates by binding to androgen receptors. This includes the activity of the accessory male sex organs and development of male secondary sex characteristics. Androgens were first discovered in 1936. Androgens are also the original anabolic steroids and the precursor of all estrogens, the female sex hormones.

Balanitis xerotica obliterans

Balanitis xerotica obliterans is a dermatological (skin) condition affecting the male genitalia. It was first described by Stuhmer in 1928, though earlier reports describe what may have been the same condition. Balanitis xerotica obliterans commonly occurs on the foreskin and glans penis.

Teratoma

A teratoma is an encapsulated tumor with tissue or organ components resembling normal derivatives of all three germ layers. There are rare occasions when not all three germ layers are identifiable. The tissues of a teratoma, although normal in themselves, may be quite different from surrounding tissues, and may be highly disparate; teratomas have been reported to contain hair, teeth, bone and, very rarely, more complex organs such as eyes, torso, and hands, feet, or other limbs.

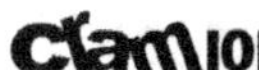

Seminoma	Seminoma (also known as pure seminoma is a germ cell tumor (cancer) of the testis. It is one of the most treatable and curable cancers, with survival >95% in the early stages. Treatment usually requires removal of one testis, but this does not affect fertility or other sexual functioning.
Penis	The penis is a biological feature of male animals including both vertebrates and invertebrates. It is a reproductive, intromittent organ that additionally serves as the urinal duct in placental mammals. Etymology The word "penis" is taken from the Latin word for "tail." Some derive that from Indo-European *pesnis, and the Greek word π?ος = "penis" from Indo-European *pesos.
Cyst	A cyst is a closed sac, having a distinct membrane and division on the nearby tissue. It may contain air, fluids, or semi-solid material. A collection of pus is called an abscess, not a cyst.
Lymphoma	Lymphoma is a cancer in the lymphatic cells of the immune system. Typically, lymphomas present as a solid tumor of lymphoid cells. Treatment might involve chemotherapy and in some cases radiotherapy and/or bone marrow transplantation, and can be curable depending on the histology, type, and stage of the disease.
Erythroplasia of Queyrat	Erythroplasia of Queyrat is a squamous cell carcinoma in situ of the glans penis. It is named for Louis Queyrat.
Systemic disease	Life-threatening disease redirects here.

	A systemic disease is one that affects a number of organs and tissues, or affects the body as a whole. Although most medical conditions will eventually involve multiple organs in advanced stage (e.g. Multiple organ dysfunction syndrome), diseases where multiple organ involvement is at presentation or in early stage are considered elsewhere.
Stoma	In botany, a stoma is a pore, found in the leaf and stem epidermis that is used for gas exchange. The pore is bordered by a pair of specialized parenchyma cells known as guard cells which are responsible for regulating the size of the opening. The term stoma is also used collectively to refer to an entire stomatal complex, both the pore itself and its accompanying guard cells.
Urinalysis	A urinalysis is an array of tests performed on urine and one of the most common methods of medical diagnosis. A part of a urinalysis can be performed by using urine dipsticks, in which the test results can be read as color changes. Medical urinalysis In addition to the substances mentioned in the table, other tests include: • a description of color and appearance. • Icotest - The test used to detect the destruction of old Red Blood Cells (RBC) in the urine. • nitrites • Hemoglobin Test - Hemolysis in the blood vessels, a rupture in the capillaries of the glomerulus, or hemorrhage in the urinary system may cause hemoglobin to appear in the urine. • hCG - normally absent, this hormone appears in the urine of pregnant women.
Urinary diversion	Urinary diversion is any one of several surgical procedures to reroute urine flow from its normal pathway. It may be necessary for diseased or defective ureters, bladder or urethra, either temporarily or permanently. Some diversions result in a stoma.

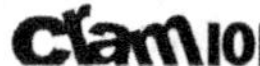

Ureterosigmoidostomy	A ureterosigmoidostomy is a surgical procedure where the ureters which carry urine from the kidneys, are diverted into the sigmoid colon. It is done as a treatment for bladder cancer, where the urinary bladder had to be removed. Rarely, the cancer presents in children between the ages of 2 ' 10 yrs old as an aggressive rhabdomyosarcoma, although there are diagnoses of children as young as 3 months old.
Pyelonephritis	Pyelonephritis is an ascending urinary tract infection that has reached the pyelum (pelvis) of the kidney . If the infection is severe, the term "urosepsis" is used interchangeably (sepsis being a systemic inflammatory response syndrome due to infection). It requires antibiotics as therapy, and treatment of any underlying causes to prevent recurrence.
Radiation	In physics, radiation describes a process in which energetic particles or waves travel through a medium or space. There are two distinct types of radiation; ionizing and non-ionizing. The word radiation is commonly used in reference to ionizing radiation only (i.e., having sufficient energy to ionize an atom), but it may also refer to non-ionizing radiation.
Radiation therapy	Radiation therapy radiation oncology, or radiotherapy (in the UK, Canada and Australia), sometimes abbreviated to XRT, is the medical use of ionizing radiation as part of cancer treatment to control malignant cells (not to be confused with radiology, the use of radiation in medical imaging and diagnosis). Radiotherapy may be used for curative or adjuvant treatment. It is used as palliative treatment (where cure is not possible and the aim is for local disease control or symptomatic relief) or as therapeutic treatment (where the therapy has survival benefit and it can be curative).
Carboplatin	Carboplatin, or cis-Diammine(1,1-cyclobutanedicarboxylato)platinum(II) is a chemotherapy drug used against some forms of cancer (mainly ovarian carcinoma, lung, head and neck cancers). It was introduced in the late 1980s and has since gained popularity in clinical treatment due to its vastly reduced side-effects compared to its parent compound cisplatin. Cisplatin and carboplatin, as well as oxaliplatin, interact with DNA, akin to the mechanism of alkylating agents.
Opioid receptor	Opioid receptors are a group of G protein-coupled receptors with opioids as ligands. The endogenous opioids are dynorphins, enkephalins, endorphins, endomorphins and nociceptin. The opioid receptors are ~40% identical to somatostatin receptors (SSTRs).
Apomorphine	Apomorphine is a non-selective dopamine agonist which activates both D_1-like and D_2-like receptors, with some preference for the latter subtypes. It is historically a morphine decomposition product by boiling with concentrated acid, hence the -morphine suffix. Apomorphine does not actually contain morphine or its skeleton, or bind to opioid receptors for that matter.

Overactive bladder	Overactive bladder is a urological condition defined by a set of symptoms: "urgency, with or without urge incontinence, usually with frequency and nocturia." Frequency is usually defined as urinating more than 8 times a day. The International Continence Society(ICS) is responsible for this definition. There exists, however, some controversy over the use of this term because these symptoms taken in isolation may overlap with those of other bladder conditions, including interstitial cystitis, or rarely even bladder tumours.
Ion channel	Ion channels are pore-forming proteins that help establish and control the small voltage gradient across the plasma membrane of cells by allowing the flow of ions down their electrochemical gradient. They are present in the membranes that surround all biological cells. The study of ion channels involves many scientific techniques such as voltage clamp electrophysiology (in particular patch clamp), immunohistochemistry, and RT-PCR. Basic features Ion channels regulate the flow of ions across the membrane in all cells.
Cystometry	Cystometry, is a clinical diagnostic procedure used to evaluate bladder function. Specifically, it measures contractile force of the bladder when voiding. The resulting chart generated from cystometric analysis is known as a cystometrogram (CMG), which plots volume of liquid emptied from bladder against intravesical pressure.
Electromyography	Electromyography is a technique for evaluating and recording the electrical activity produced by skeletal muscles. EMG is performed using an instrument called an electromyograph, to produce a record called an electromyogram. An electromyograph detects the electrical potential generated by muscle cells when these cells are electrically or neurologically activated.
Spinal shock	Spinal shock was first defined by Whytt in 1750 as a loss of sensation accompanied by motor paralysis with initial loss but gradual recovery of reflexes, following a spinal cord injury (SCI) - most often a complete transection. Reflexes in the spinal cord caudal to the SCI are depressed (hyporeflexia) or absent (areflexia), while those rostral to the SCI remain unaffected. Note that the 'shock' in spinal shock does not refer to circulatory collapse.

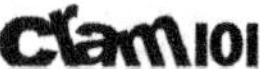

Feedback	Feedback describes the situation when output from (or information about the result of) an event or phenomenon in the past will influence an occurrence or occurrences of the same (i.e. same defined) event / phenomenon (or the continuation / development of the original phenomenon) in the present or future. When an event is part of a chain of cause-and-effect that forms a circuit or loop, then the event is said to "feed back" into itself. Feedback is also a synonym for: • Feedback signal - the information about the initial event that is the basis for subsequent modification of the event • Feedback loop - the causal path that leads from the initial generation of the feedback signal to the subsequent modification of the event • Audio feedback - the special kind of positive feedback that occurs when a loop exists between an audio input and output. Overview Feedback is a mechanism, process or signal that is looped back to control a system within itself.
Autonomic dysreflexia	Autonomic dysreflexia, "Autonomic dysreflexia" also known as "autonomic hyperreflexia or Hyperreflexia, is a potentially life threatening condition which can be considered a medical emergency requiring immediate attention. Autonomic dysreflexia occurs most often in spinal cord-injured individuals with spinal lesions above the (T6) spinal cord level. Acute Autonomic dysreflexia is a reaction of the autonomic (involuntary) nervous system to overstimulation.
Interstitial cystitis	Interstitial cystitis is a chronic, severely debilitating disease of the urinary bladder. Of unknown cause, it is characterised by: pain associated with the bladder, pain associated with urination (dysuria), urinary frequency (as often as every 10 minutes), urgency, and/or pressure in the bladder and/or pelvis. The disease has a profound impact on quality of life.

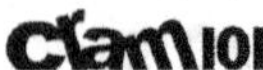

Enuresis	Enuresis refers to an inability to control urination. Use of the term is usually limited to describing individuals old enough to be expected to exercise such control. Types of enuresis include: • Nocturnal enuresis • Diurnal enuresis The controversial diagnosis PANDAS (pediatric autoimmune neuropsychiatric disorders associated with streptococcal infections) has been used to describe a set of children who have a rapid onset of OCD and/or tic disorders following a streptococcal infection, with a link to other symptoms such as enuresis.
Spina bifida	Spina bifida is a developmental congenital disorder caused by the incomplete closing of the embryonic neural tube. Some vertebrae overlying the spinal cord are not fully formed and remain unfused and open. If the opening is large enough, this allows a portion of the spinal cord to protrude through the opening in the bones.
Nephropathy	Nephropathy refers to damage to or disease of the kidney. An older term for this is nephrosis. Causes of nephropathy include administration of analgesics, xanthine oxidase deficiency, and long-term exposure to lead or its salts.
Nifedipine	Nifedipine is a dihydropyridine calcium channel blocker. Its main uses are as an antianginal (especially in Prinzmetal's angina) and antihypertensive, although a large number of other indications have recently been found for this agent, such as Raynaud's phenomenon, premature labor, and painful spasms of the esophagus in cancer and tetanus patients. It is also commonly used for the small subset of pulmonary hypertension patients whose symptoms respond to calcium channel blockers.
Sexual dysfunction	Sexual dysfunction, including desire, arousal or orgasm.

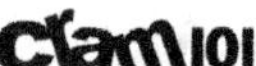

To maximize the benefits of medications and behavioural techniques in the management of sexual dysfunction it is important to have a comprehensive approach to the problem,A thorough sexual history and assessment of general health and other sexual problems (if any) are very important. Assessing (performance) anxiety, guilt (associated with masturbation in many South-Asian men), stress and worry are integral to the optimal management of sexual dysfunction.

Nomenclature

Nomenclature is a term that applies to either a list of names and/or terms, or to the system of principles, procedures and terms related to naming - which is the assigning of a word or phrase to a particular object or property. The principles of naming vary from the relatively informal conventions of everyday speech to the internationally-agreed principles, rules and recommendations that govern the formation and use of the specialist terms used in scientific and other disciplines.

Naming "things" is a part of our general communication using words and language: it is an aspect of everyday taxonomy as we distinguish the objects of our experience, together with their similarities and differences, which we identify, name and classify.

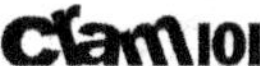

Urinary incontinence	Urinary incontinence is any involuntary leakage of urine. It is a common and distressing problem, which may have a profound impact on quality of life. Urinary incontinence almost always results from an underlying treatable medical condition but is under-reported to medical practitioners.
Pathophysiology	Pathophysiology is the study of the changes of normal mechanical, physical, and biochemical functions, either caused by a disease, or resulting from an abnormal syndrome. More formally, it is the branch of medicine which deals with any disturbances of body functions, caused by disease or prodromal symptoms. An alternative definition is "the study of the biological and physical manifestations of disease as they correlate with the underlying abnormalities and physiological disturbances." The study of pathology and the study of pathophysiology often involves substantial overlap in diseases and processes, but pathology emphasizes direct observations, while pathophysiology emphasizes quantifiable measurements.
Anatomy	Anatomy is a branch of biology and medicine that is the consideration of the structure of living things. It is a general term that includes human anatomy, animal anatomy and plant anatomy. In some of its facets anatomy is closely related to embryology, comparative anatomy and comparative embryology, through common roots in evolution.
Cystography	In radiology and urology, a cystography is a procedure used to visualise the urinary bladder. Using an urinary catheter, radiocontrast is instilled in the bladder, and X-ray imaging is performed. Cystography can be used to evaluate bladder cancer, vesicoureteral reflux, bladder polyps, and hydronephrosis.
Diagnosis	Diagnosis is the identification of the nature and cause of anything. Diagnosis is used in many different disciplines with variations in the use of logics, analytics, and experience to determine the cause and effect relationships. In systems engineering and computer science, diagnosis is typically used to determine the causes of symptoms, mitigations for problems, and solutions to issues.

Urge incontinence	Urge incontinence is a form of urinary incontinence. Urge incontinence is involuntary loss of urine occurring for no apparent reason while feeling urinary urgency, a sudden need or urge to urinate. The most common cause of urge incontinence is involuntary and inappropriate detrusor muscle contractions.
Adenocarcinoma	Adenocarcinoma is a cancer of an epithelium that originates in glandular tissue. Epithelial tissue includes, but is not limited to, the surface layer of skin, glands and a variety of other tissue that lines the cavities and organs of the body. Epithelium can be derived embryologically from ectoderm, endoderm or mesoderm.
Pathology	Pathology is the study and diagnosis of disease. The word pathology is from Greek π?θος, pathos, "feeling, suffering"; and -λογ?α, -logia, "the study of". Pathologization, to pathologize, refers to the process of defining a condition or behavior as pathological, e.g. pathological gambling.
Symptom	A symptom is a departure from normal function or feeling which is noticed by a patient, indicating the presence of disease or abnormality. A symptom is subjective, observed by the patient, and not measured. A symptom may not be a malady, for example symptoms of pregnancy.

Laboratory

A laboratory is a facility that provides controlled conditions in which scientific research, experiments, and measurement may be performed. The title of laboratory is also used for certain other facilities where the processes or equipment used are similar to those in scientific laboratories. These notably include:

- the film laboratory or darkroom
- the computer lab
- the medical lab
- the public health lab
- the clandestine lab for the production of illegal drugs

In recent years government and private centers for innovation in learning, leadership and organization have adopted "lab" in their name to emphasize the experimental and research-oriented nature of their work.

Electromyography

Electromyography is a technique for evaluating and recording the electrical activity produced by skeletal muscles. EMG is performed using an instrument called an electromyograph, to produce a record called an electromyogram. An electromyograph detects the electrical potential generated by muscle cells when these cells are electrically or neurologically activated.

Radiography

Radiography is the use of X-rays to view a non uniformly composed material such as the human body. By utilizing the physical properties of the ray an image can be developed displaying clearly, areas of different density and composition.

A heterogeneous beam of X-rays is produced by an X-ray generator and is projected toward an object.

Adrenalectomy

Adrenalectomy is the surgical removal of one or both (bilateral adrenalectomy) adrenal glands. It is usually advised for patients with tumors of the adrenal glands. The procedure can be performed using an open incision or laparoscopic technique.

Intersex	Intersex in humans refers to intermediate or atypical combinations of physical features that usually distinguish female from male. This is usually understood to be congenital, involving chromosomal, morphologic, genital and/or gonadal anomalies, such as diversion from typical XX-female or XY-male presentations, e.g., sex reversal (XY-female, XX-male), genital ambiguity, sex developmental differences. An intersex individual may have biological characteristics of both the male and the female sexes.
Mitosis	Mitosis is the process by which a eukaryotic cell separates the chromosomes in its cell nucleus into two identical sets in two nuclei. It is generally followed immediately by cytokinesis, which divides the nuclei, cytoplasm, organelles and cell membrane into two cells containing roughly equal shares of these cellular components. Mitosis and cytokinesis together define the mitotic (M) phase of the cell cycle--the division of the mother cell into two daughter cells, genetically identical to each other and to their parent cell.
Pseudohermaphroditism	Pseudohermaphroditism, is the condition in which an organism is born with secondary sex characteristics or a phenotype that is different from what would be expected on the basis of the gonadal tissue (ovary or testis). In some cases, the external sex organs look intermediate between the typical clitoris or penis. In other cases, the external sex organs have an appearance that does not look intermediate, but rather has the appearance that would be expected to be seen with the "opposite" gonadal tissue.
Congenital adrenal hyperplasia	Congenital adrenal hyperplasia refers to any of several autosomal recessive diseases resulting from mutations of genes for enzymes mediating the biochemical steps of production of cortisol from cholesterol by the adrenal glands (steroidogenesis). congenital adrenal hyperplasia is one of the possible underlying synthesis problems in Addison's disease. Most of these conditions involve excessive or deficient production of sex steroids and can alter development of primary or secondary sex characteristics in some affected infants, children, or adults.

Prognosis	Prognosis is a medical term to describe the likely outcome of an illness. When applied to large populations, prognostic estimates can be very accurate: for example the statement "45% of patients with severe septic shock will die within 28 days" can be made with some confidence, because previous research found that this proportion of patients died. However, it is much harder to translate this into a prognosis for an individual patient: additional information is needed to determine whether a patient belongs to the 45% who will succumb, or to the 55% who survive.
Urethritis	Urethritis is inflammation of the urethra. The main symptom is dysuria, which is painful or difficult urination. The disease is classified as either gonococcocal urethritis, caused by Neisseria gonorrhoeae, or non-gonococcal urethritis most commonly caused by Chlamydia trachomatis.
Pheochromocytoma	A pheochromocytoma is a neuroendocrine tumor of the medulla of the adrenal glands (originating in the chromaffin cells), or extra-adrenal chromaffin tissue that failed to involute after birth and secretes excessive amounts of catecholamines, usually adrenaline (epinephrine) if in the adrenal gland and not extra-adrenal, and noradrenaline (norepinephrine). Extra-adrenal paragangliomas (often described as extra-adrenal pheochromocytomas) are closely related, though less common, tumors that originate in the ganglia of the sympathetic nervous system and are named based upon the primary anatomical site of origin. Signs and symptoms

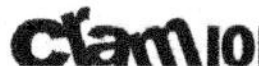

The signs and symptoms of a pheochromocytoma are those of sympathetic nervous system hyperactivity, including:

- Skin sensations
- Flank pain
- Elevated heart rate
- Elevated blood pressure, including paroxysmal (sporadic, episodic) high blood pressure, which sometimes can be more difficult to detect; another clue to the presence of pheochromocytoma is orthostatic hypotension (a fall in systolic blood pressure greater than 20 mmHg or a fall in diastolic blood pressure greater than 10 mmHg on making the patient stand)
- Palpitations
- Anxiety often resembling that of a panic attack
- Diaphoresis (excessive sweating)
- Headaches
- Pallor
- Weight loss
- Localized amyloid deposits found microscopically
- Elevated blood glucose level (due primarily to catecholamine stimulation of lipolysis (breakdown of stored fat) leading to high levels of free fatty acids and the subsequent inhibition of glucose uptake by muscle cells.

Tumor

A tumor is the name for a neoplasm or a solid lesion formed by an abnormal growth of cells (termed neoplastic) which looks like a swelling. Tumor is not synonymous with cancer. A tumor can be benign, pre-malignant or malignant, whereas cancer is by definition malignant.

Urine

Urine is a sterile (in the absence of a disease condition), liquid by-product of the body that is secreted by the kidneys through a process called urination and excreted through the urethra. Cellular metabolism generates numerous by-products, many rich in nitrogen, that require elimination from the bloodstream. These by-products are eventually expelled from the body in a process known as micturition, the primary method for excreting water-soluble chemicals from the body.

Differential diagnosis

A differential diagnosis is a systematic method used to identify unknowns. This method, essentially a process of elimination, is used by taxonomists to identify living organisms, and by physicians, nurse practitioners, physician assistants, and other trained medical professionals to diagnose the specific disease in a patient.

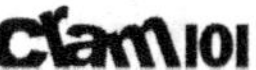

Not all medical diagnoses are differential ones: some diagnoses merely name a set of signs and symptoms that may have more than one possible cause, and some diagnoses are based on intuition or estimations of likelihood.

Lymphoma

Lymphoma is a cancer in the lymphatic cells of the immune system. Typically, lymphomas present as a solid tumor of lymphoid cells. Treatment might involve chemotherapy and in some cases radiotherapy and/or bone marrow transplantation, and can be curable depending on the histology, type, and stage of the disease.

Agenesis

In medicine, agenesis refers to the failure of an organ to develop during embryonic growth and development. Many forms of agenesis are referred to by individual names, depending on the organ affected:

- Agenesis of the corpus callosum- failure of the Corpus callosum to develop
- Renal agenesis- failure of one or both of the kidneys to develop
- Phocomelia- failure of the arms or legs to develop
- Penile agenesis- failure of penis to develop
- Müllerian agenesis - failure of the uterus and part of the vagina to develop

Eye agenesis

Eye agenesis is a medical condition in which sufferers are born with no eyes.

Dental ' oral agenesis

- anodontia
- aglossia
- agnathia

Ear agenesis

Ear agenesis is a medical condition in which people are born without ears.

Kidney	The kidneys are organs with several functions. They are seen in many types of animals, including vertebrates and some invertebrates. They are an essential part of the urinary system and also serve homeostatic functions such as the regulation of electrolytes, maintenance of acid-base balance, and regulation of blood pressure.
Renal agenesis	Renal agenesis is a unilateral or bilateral medical condition in which fetal kidneys fail to develop leading to oligohydramnios, resulting in a 40-fold increase in perinatal mortality. It can be associated with RET or UPK3A. Bilateral Bilateral renal agenesis is the uncommon and serious failure of both a fetus' kidneys to develop during gestation, and is one causative agent of Potter sequence. This absence of kidneys causes oligohydramnios, a deficiency of amniotic fluid in a pregnant woman, which can place extra pressure on the developing baby and cause further malformations.
Renal failure	Renal failure or kidney failure (formerly called renal insufficiency) describes a medical condition in which the kidneys fail to adequately filter toxins and waste products from the blood. The two forms are acute (acute kidney injury) and chronic (chronic kidney disease); a number of other diseases or health problems may cause either form of renal failure to occur. Renal failure is described as a decrease in the glomerular filtration rate.
Supernumerary kidney	A supernumerary kidney is an additional kidney to the number usually present in an organism. This often develops as the result of splitting of the nephrogenic blastema, or from separate metanephric blastemas into which partially or completely reduplicated ureteral stalks enter to form separate capsulated kidneys; in some cases the separation of the reduplicated organ is incomplete (fused supernumerary kidney).
Cyst	A cyst is a closed sac, having a distinct membrane and division on the nearby tissue. It may contain air, fluids, or semi-solid material. A collection of pus is called an abscess, not a cyst.

Polycystic kidney disease	Polycystic Kidney Disease is a cystic genetic disorder of the kidneys. There are two types of Polycystic kidney disease: Autosomal Dominant Polycystic Kidney Disease and the less-common Autosomal Recessive Polycystic Kidney Disease. It occurs in humans and some other animals.
Etiology	Etiology is the study of causation, or origination. The word is most commonly used in medical and philosophical theories, where it is used to refer to the study of why things occur, or even the reasons behind the way that things act, and is used in philosophy, physics, psychology, government, medicine, theology and biology in reference to the causes of various phenomena. An etiological myth is a myth intended to explain a name or create a mythic history for a place or family.
Tuberous sclerosis	Tuberous sclerosis is a rare, multi-system genetic disease that causes non-malignant tumors to grow in the brain and on other vital organs such as the kidneys, heart, eyes, lungs, and skin. A combination of symptoms may include seizures, developmental delay, behavioral problems, skin abnormalities, lung and kidney disease. TSC is caused by a mutation of either of two genes, TSC1 and TSC2, which encode for the proteins hamartin and tuberin respectively.
Reflux	Reflux is a technique involving the condensation of vapors and the return of this condensate to the system from which it originated. It is used in industrial and laboratory distillations. It is also used in chemistry to supply energy to reactions over a long period of time.
Vesicoureteral reflux	Vesicoureteral reflux is an abnormal movement of urine from the bladder into ureters or kidneys. Urine normally travels from the kidneys via the ureters to the bladder. In vesicoureteral reflux the direction of urine flow is reversed (retrograde).
Voiding cystourethrogram	In urology, a voiding cystourethrogram also micturating cystourethrogram (MCUG), is a technique for watching a person's urethra and urinary bladder while the person urinates (voids). The technique consists of catheterizing the person in order to fill the bladder with a radiopaque liquid (a "contrast" or "contrast agent", typically cystografin). Under fluoroscopy (real time x-rays) the radiologist watches the contrast enter the bladder and looks at the anatomy of the patient.

Renal cyst	A renal cyst is a fluid collection in the kidney. There are several types based on the Bosniak classification. The majority are benign, simple cysts that can be monitored and not intervened upon.
Echinococcosis	Echinococcosis, which is often times referred to as hydatid disease or echinococcal disease, is a parasitic disease that affects both humans and other mammals, such as sheep, dogs, rodents and horses. There are three different forms of echinococcosis found in humans, each of which is caused by the larval stages of different species of the tapeworm of genus Echinococcus. The first of the three and also the most common form found in humans is cystic echinococcosis which is caused by Echinococcus granulosus.
Medullary sponge kidney	Also known as Cacchi Ricci disease, medullary sponge kidney is a congenital disorder of the kidneys characterized by cystic dilatation of the collecting tubules in one or both kidneys. It has been estimated to occur with a frequency of 1 in every 5,000 individuals in a population. The disease is bilateral in 70% of cases.
Renal vein thrombosis	Renal vein thrombosis is the formation of a clot or thrombus obstructing the renal vein, leading to a reduction in drainage of the kidney. Presentation This thrombosis can lead to imbalances in blood clotting factor. Its symptoms may include blood in urine or being diminished in volume.
Angiomyolipoma	Angiomyolipoma are the most common benign tumour of the kidney and are composed of blood vessels, smooth muscle cells and fat cells. Angiomyolipoma are strongly associated with the genetic disease tuberous sclerosis, in which most individuals will have several angiomyolipoma affecting both kidneys. They are also commonly found in women with the rare lung disease lymphangioleiomyomatosis.
Urination	Urination, voiding, peeing, weeing, pissing, and more rarely, emiction, is the ejection of urine from the urinary bladder through the urethra to the outside of the body. In healthy humans the process of urination is under voluntary control. In infants, elderly individuals and those with neurological injury, urination may occur as an involuntary reflex.

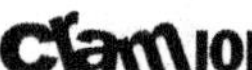

Cancer	Cancer (medical term: malignant neoplasm) is a class of diseases in which a group of cells display uncontrolled growth, invasion that intrudes upon and destroys adjacent tissues, and sometimes metastasis, or spreading to other locations in the body via lymph or blood. These three malignant properties of cancers differentiate them from benign tumors, which do not invade or metastasize. Researchers divide the causes of cancer into two groups: those with an environmental cause and those with a hereditary genetic cause.
Carcinoma	Carcinoma is the medical condition of an invasive malignant tumor consisting of transformed epithelial cells. Alternatively, it refers to a malignant tumor composed of transformed cells of unknown histogenesis, but which possess specific molecular or histological characteristics that are associated with epithelial cells, such as the production of cytokeratins or intercellular bridges.
Physical examination	Physical examination is the process by which a doctor investigates the body of a patient for signs of disease. It generally follows the taking of the medical history -- an account of the symptoms as experienced by the patient. Together with the medical history, the physical examination aids in determining the correct diagnosis and devising the treatment plan.
Prostate	The prostate is a compound tubuloalveolar exocrine gland of the male reproductive system in most mammals. In 2002, female paraurethral glands, or Skene's glands, were officially renamed the female prostate by the Federative International Committee on Anatomical Terminology. The prostate differs considerably among species anatomically, chemically, and physiologically.
Prostate cancer	Prostate cancer is a form of cancer that develops in the prostate, a gland in the male reproductive system. Most prostate cancers are slow growing; however, there are cases of aggressive prostate cancers. The cancer cells may metastasize (spread) from the prostate to other parts of the body, particularly the bones and lymph nodes.

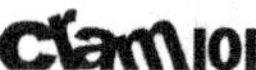

Renal biopsy	A renal biopsy is a procedure in which a sample of kidney (also called renal) tissue is obtained. Microscopic examination of the tissue can provide information needed to diagnose, monitor or treat a renal disorder. Indications Renal biopsy is recommended for selected patients with kidney disease.
Glomerulonephritis	Glomerulonephritis, abbreviated GN, is a renal disease (usually of both kidneys) characterized by inflammation of the glomeruli, or small blood vessels in the kidneys. It may present with isolated hematuria and/or proteinuria (blood or protein in the urine); or as a nephrotic syndrome, a nephritic syndrome, acute renal failure, or chronic renal failure. They are categorised into several different pathological patterns, which are broadly grouped into non-proliferative or proliferative types.
IgA nephropathy	IgA nephropathy is a form of glomerulonephritis (inflammation of the glomeruli of the kidney). This should not be confused with Buerger's disease, an unrelated condition. IgA nephropathy is the most common glomerulonephritis throughout the world Primary IgA nephropathy is characterized by deposition of the IgA antibody in the glomerulus.
Nephropathy	Nephropathy refers to damage to or disease of the kidney. An older term for this is nephrosis. Causes of nephropathy include administration of analgesics, xanthine oxidase deficiency, and long-term exposure to lead or its salts.
Germ cell	A germ cell is any biological cell that gives rise to the gametes of an organism that reproduces sexually. In many animals, the germ cells originate near the gut of an embryo and migrate to the developing gonads. There, they undergo cell division of two types, mitosis and meiosis, followed by cellular differentiation into mature gametes, either eggs or sperm.

Toxicity	Toxicity is the degree to which a substance can damage an organism. Toxicity can refer to the effect on a whole organism, such as an animal, bacterium, or plant, as well as the effect on a substructure of the organism, such as a cell (cytotoxicity) or an organ (organotoxicity), such as the liver (hepatotoxicity). By extension, the word may be metaphorically used to describe toxic effects on larger and more complex groups, such as the family unit or society at large.
Nephrotic syndrome	Nephrotic syndrome is a nonspecific disorder in which the kidneys are damaged, causing them to leak large amounts of protein (proteinuria at least 3.5 grams per day per 1.73m^2 body surface area) from the blood into the urine. Kidneys affected by nephrotic syndrome have small pores in the podocytes, large enough to permit proteinuria (and subsequently hypoalbuminemia, because some of the protein albumin has gone from the blood to the urine) but not large enough to allow cells through (hence no hematuria). By contrast, in nephritic syndrome, RBCs pass through the pores, causing hematuria.
Oliguria	Oliguria is the low output of urine, It is clinically classified as an output below 400 ml/day . The decreased output of urine may be a sign of dehydration, renal failure, hypovolemic shock, multiple organ dysfunction syndrome, or urinary obstruction/urinary retention. It can be contrasted with anuria, which represents an absence of urine, clinically classified as below 50ml/day.
Epididymitis	Epididymitis is a medical condition in which there is inflammation of the epididymis (a curved structure at the back of the testicle in which sperm matures and is stored). This condition may be mildly to very painful, and the scrotum (sac containing the testicles) may become red, warm and swollen. It may be acute (of sudden onset) or rarely chronic.
Glomerulosclerosis	Glomerulosclerosis refers to a hardening of the glomerulus in the kidney. It is a general term to describe scarring of the kidneys' tiny blood vessels, the glomeruli, the functional units in the kidney that filter urine from the blood

Proteinuria (large amounts of protein in urine) is one of the signs of glomerulosclerosis. Scarring disturbs the filtering process of the kidneys and allows protein to leak from the blood into urine.

Membranoproliferative glomerulonephritis

Membranoproliferative glomerulonephritis also known as mesangiocapillary glomerulonephritis, is a type of glomerulonephritis caused by deposits in the kidney glomerular mesangium and basement membrane (GBM) thickening, activating complement and damaging the glomeruli.

MPGN accounts for approximately 4% of primary renal causes of nephrotic syndrome in children and 7% in adults.

It should not be confused with membranous glomerulonephritis, a condition in where the basement membrane is thickened, but the mesangium is not.

Analgesic nephropathy

Analgesic nephropathy is injury to the kidney caused by analgesic medications such as aspirin, phenacetin, and paracetamol. The term usually refers to damage induced by excessive use of combinations of these medications, especially combinations that include phenacetin. It may also be used to describe kidney injury from any single analgesic medication.

Collagen disease

Collagen disease is a term previously used to describe systemic autoimmune diseases (e.g., rheumatoid arthritis, systemic lupus erythematosus, and systemic sclerosis), but now is thought to be more appropriate for diseases associated with defects in collagen, which is a component of the connective tissue.

The term "collagen disease" was coined by Dr. Paul Klemperer at Mount Sinai Hospital in New York City in 1941.

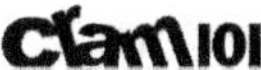

Interstitial nephritis	Interstitial nephritis is a form of nephritis affecting the interstitium of the kidneys surrounding the tubules. This disease can be either acute, meaning it occurs suddenly, or chronic, meaning it is ongoing and eventually ends in kidney failure. Etiologies Common causes include infection, or reaction to medication (such as an analgesic or antibiotics such as methicillin).
Nephritis	Nephritis is inflammation of the nephrons in the kidneys. The word "nephritis" was imported from Latin, which took it from Greek: νεφρ?τιδα. The word comes from the Greek νεφρ?ς - nephro- meaning "of the kidney" and -itis meaning "inflammation".
Pyelonephritis	Pyelonephritis is an ascending urinary tract infection that has reached the pyelum (pelvis) of the kidney . If the infection is severe, the term "urosepsis" is used interchangeably (sepsis being a systemic inflammatory response syndrome due to infection). It requires antibiotics as therapy, and treatment of any underlying causes to prevent recurrence.
Uric acid	Uric acid is a heterocyclic compound of carbon, nitrogen, oxygen, and hydrogen with the formula $C_5H_4N_4O_3$. Uric acid is created when the body breaks down purine nucleotides. Chemistry Uric acid is a diprotic acid with pKa_1=5.4 and pKa_2=10.3. Thus in strong alkali at high pH, it forms the dually charged full urate ion, but at biological pH or in the presence of carbonic acid or carbonate ions, it forms the singly charged hydrogen or acid urate ion as its pKa_2 is greater than the pKa_1 of carbonic acid.

Cystitis	Cystitis is a term that refers to urinary bladder inflammation that results from any one of a number of distinct syndromes . It is most commonly caused by a bacterial infection in which case it is referred to as a urinary tract infection. Signs and symptoms • Pressure in the lower pelvis • Painful urination (dysuria) • Frequent urination (polyuria) or urgent need to urinate (urinary urgency) • Need to urinate at night (nocturia, similar to prostate cancer or BPH) • Abnormal urine color (cloudy), similar to a urinary tract infection • Foul or strong urine odor Differential diagnosis There are several medically distinct types of cystitis, each having a unique etiology and therapeutic approach: • Traumatic cystitis is probably the most common form of cystitis in the female, and is due to bruising of the bladder, usually by abnormally forceful sexual intercourse.
Fanconi syndrome	Fanconi syndrome is a disease of the proximal renal tubules of the kidney in which glucose, amino acids, uric acid, phosphate and bicarbonate are passed into the urine, instead of being reabsorbed. Fanconi syndrome affects the proximal tubule, which is the first part of the tubule to process fluid after it is filtered through the glomerulus. It may be inherited, or caused by drugs or heavy metals.
Glycosuria	Glycosuria is the excretion of glucose into the urine. Ordinarily, urine contains no glucose because the kidneys are able to reclaim all of the filtered glucose back into the bloodstream. Glycosuria is nearly always caused by elevated blood glucose levels, most commonly due to untreated diabetes mellitus.

Renal tubular acidosis	Renal tubular acidosis is a medical condition that involves an accumulation of acid in the body due to a failure of the kidneys to appropriately acidify the urine. When blood is filtered by the kidney, the filtrate passes through the tubules of the nephron, allowing for exchange of salts, acid equivalents, and other solutes before it drains into the bladder as urine. The metabolic acidosis that results from Renal tubular acidosis may be caused either by failure to recover sufficient (alkaline) bicarbonate ions from the filtrate in the early portion of the nephron (proximal tubule) or by insufficient secretion of (acid) hydrogen ions into the latter portions of the nephron (distal tubule).
Nephrocalcinosis	Nephrocalcinosis, once known as Albright's calcinosis after Fuller Albright, is a term originally used to describe deposition of calcium salts in the renal parenchyma due to hyperparathyroidism. It is now more commonly used to describe diffuse, fine, renal parenchymal calcification on radiology. During its early stages, nephrocalcinosis is visible on x-ray, and appears as a fine granular mottling over the renal outlines.
Sodium	Sodium is a metallic element with a symbol Na and atomic number 11. It is a soft, silvery-white, highly reactive metal and is a member of the alkali metals within "group 1" (formerly known as 'group IA'). It has only one stable isotope, ^{23}Na. Elemental sodium was first isolated by Humphry Davy in 1807 by passing an electric current through molten sodium hydroxide.
Vascular	Vascular in zoology and medicine means "related to blood vessels", which are part of the circulatory system. An organ or tissue that is vascularized is heavily endowed with blood vessels and thus richly supplied with blood. In botany, plants with a dedicated transport system for water and nutrients are called vascular plants.
Hemodialysis	In medicine, hemodialysis is a method for removing waste products such as creatinine and urea, as well as free water from the blood when the kidneys are in renal failure. Hemodialysis is one of three renal replacement therapies (the other two being renal transplant; peritoneal dialysis).

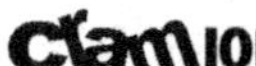

	Hemodialysis can be an outpatient or inpatient therapy.
Peritoneal dialysis	Peritoneal dialysis is a treatment for patients with severe chronic kidney disease. The process uses the patient's peritoneum in the abdomen as a membrane across which fluids and dissolved substances (electrolytes, urea, glucose, albumin and other small molecules) are exchanged from the blood. Fluid is introduced through a permanent tube in the abdomen and flushed out either every night while the patient sleeps (automatic peritoneal dialysis) or via regular exchanges throughout the day (continuous ambulatory peritoneal dialysis).
Nephrectomy	Nephrectomy is the surgical removal of a kidney. History The first successful nephrectomy was performed by the German surgeon Gustav Simon on August 2, 1869 in Heidelberg. Simon practiced the operation beforehand in animal experiments.
Infection	An infection is the colonization of a host organism by parasite species. Infecting parasites seek to use the host's resources to reproduce, often resulting in disease. Colloquially, infections are usually considered to be caused by microscopic organisms or microparasites like viruses, prions, bacteria, and viroids, though larger organisms like macroparasites and fungi can also infect.
Infection	An infection is the colonization of a host organism by parasite species. Infecting parasites seek to use the host's resources to reproduce, often resulting in disease. Colloquially, infections are usually considered to be caused by microscopic organisms or microparasites like viruses, prions, bacteria, and viroids, though larger organisms like macroparasites and fungi can also infect.
Erectile dysfunction	Erectile dysfunction is sexual dysfunction characterized by the inability to develop or maintain an erection of the penis during sexual performance.

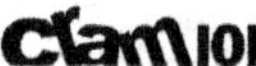

A penile erection is the hydraulic effect of blood entering and being retained in sponge-like bodies within the penis. The process is often initiated as a result of sexual arousal, when signals are transmitted from the brain to nerves in the penis.

Risk factor

In epidemiology, a risk factor is a variable associated with an increased risk of disease or infection. Sometimes, determinant is also used, being a variable associated with either increased or decreased risk. Risk factors or determinants are correlational and not necessarily causal, because correlation does not imply causation.

Blood transfusion

Blood transfusion is the process of transferring blood or blood-based products from one person into the circulatory system of another. Blood transfusions can be life-saving in some situations, such as massive blood loss due to trauma, or can be used to replace blood lost during surgery. Blood transfusions may also be used to treat a severe anaemia or thrombocytopenia caused by a blood disease.

Bladder cancer

Bladder cancer refers to any of several types of malignant growths of the urinary bladder. It is a disease in which abnormal cells multiply without control in the bladder. The bladder is a hollow, muscular organ that stores urine; it is located in the pelvis.

Cross-matching

Cross-matching blood, in transfusion medicine, refers to the complex testing that is performed prior to a blood transfusion, to determine if the donor's blood is compatible with the blood of an intended recipient, or to identify matches for organ transplants. Cross-matching is usually performed only after other, less complex tests have not excluded compatibility. Blood compatibility has many aspects, and is determined not only by the blood types (O, A, B, AB), but also by blood factors, (Rh, Kell, etc)..

Tissue typing

Tissue typing is a procedure in which the tissues of a prospective donor and recipient are tested for compatibility prior to transplantation. An embryo can be tissue typed to ensure that the embryo implanted can be a cord-blood stem cell donor for a sick sibling.

One technique of tissue typing, "mixed leukocyte reaction", is performed by culturing lymphocytes from the donor together with those from the recipient.

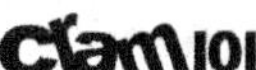

Corticosteroid	Corticosteroids are a class of steroid hormones that are produced in the adrenal cortex. Corticosteroids are involved in a wide range of physiologic systems such as stress response, immune response and regulation of inflammation, carbohydrate metabolism, protein catabolism, blood electrolyte levels, and behavior. • Glucocorticoids such as cortisol control carbohydrate, fat and protein metabolism and are anti-inflammatory by preventing phospholipid release, decreasing eosinophil action and a number of other mechanisms. • Mineralocorticoids such as aldosterone control electrolyte and water levels, mainly by promoting sodium retention in the kidney. Some common natural hormones are corticosterone ($C_{21}H_{30}O_4$), cortisone ($C_{21}H_{28}O_5$, 17-hydroxy-11-dehydrocorticosterone) and aldosterone.
Immunosuppressive drug	Immunosuppressive drugs or immunosuppressive agents are drugs that inhibit or prevent activity of the immune system. They are used in immunosuppressive therapy to: • Prevent the rejection of transplanted organs and tissues (e.g., bone marrow, heart, kidney, liver) • Treat autoimmune diseases or diseases that are most likely of autoimmune origin (e.g., rheumatoid arthritis, multiple sclerosis, myasthenia gravis, systemic lupus erythematosus, focal segmental glomerulosclerosis, Crohn's disease, Behcet's Disease, pemphigus, and ulcerative colitis). • Treat some other non-autoimmune inflammatory diseases (e.g., long term allergic asthma control). These drugs are not without side-effects and risks. Because the majority of them act non-selectively, the immune system is less able to resist infections and the spread of malignant cells.
Infertility	Infertility primarily refers to the biological inability of a person to contribute to conception. Infertility may also refer to the state of a woman who is unable to carry a pregnancy to full term. There are many biological causes of infertility, some which may be bypassed with medical intervention.

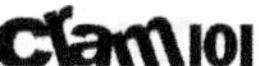

Azathioprine	Azathioprine is a drug that suppresses the immune system. Azathioprine is used in organ transplantation and autoimmune disease. Some of the autoimmune diseases are rheumatoid arthritis, pemphigus, Inflammatory Bowel Disease (such as Crohn's disease and Ulcerative Colitis), multiple sclerosis, autoimmune hepatitis, atopic dermatitis, Myasthenia Gravis, Neuromyelitis Optica and restrictive lung disease.
Leflunomide	Leflunomide is a medication of the DMARD type, used in active moderate to severe rheumatoid arthritis and psoriatic arthritis. It is a pyrimidine synthesis inhibitor. Basic chemical, pharmacological, and marketing data Leflunomide is a pyrimidine synthesis inhibitor belonging to the DMARD (disease-modifying antirheumatic drug) class of drugs, which are chemically and pharmacologically very heterogeneous.
Mycophenolate mofetil	Mycophenolate mofetil(CellCept by Roche) is a immunosuppressant and prodrug of mycophenolic acid, used extensively in transplant medicine. Its mode of action is as a reversible inhibitor of inosine monophosphate dehydrogenase (IMPDH) in purine biosynthesis. MMF is selective for the de novo pathway critical to lymphocytic proliferation and activation.
Tuberculosis	Tuberculosis, MTB or TB (short for tubercles bacillus) is a common and in some cases deadly infectious disease caused by various strains of mycobacteria, usually Mycobacterium tuberculosis in humans. Tuberculosis usually attacks the lungs but can also affect other parts of the body. It is spread through the air when people who have active MTB infection cough, sneeze, or spit.
Cyclophosphamide	Cyclophosphamide also known as cytophosphane, is a nitrogen mustard alkylating agent, from the oxazophorines group. An alkylating agent adds an alkyl group (C_nH_{2n+1}) to DNA. It attaches the alkyl group to the guanine base of DNA, at the number 7 nitrogen atom of the imidazole ring.

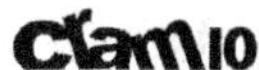

	It is used to treat various types of cancer and some autoimmune disorders.
Polyclonal antibodies	Polyclonal antibodies are antibodies that are obtained from different B cell resources. They are a combination of immunoglobulin molecules secreted against a specific antigen, each identifying a different epitope. Production These antibodies are typically produced by immunization of a suitable mammal, such as a mouse, rabbit or goat.
Monoclonal antibodies	Monoclonal antibodies are monospecific antibodies that are the same because they are made by identical immune cells that are all clones of a unique parent cell. Given almost any substance, it is possible to produce monoclonal antibodies that specifically bind to that substance; they can then serve to detect or purify that substance. This has become an important tool in biochemistry, molecular biology and medicine.
Cancer	Cancer (medical term: malignant neoplasm) is a class of diseases in which a group of cells display uncontrolled growth, invasion that intrudes upon and destroys adjacent tissues, and sometimes metastasis, or spreading to other locations in the body via lymph or blood. These three malignant properties of cancers differentiate them from benign tumors, which do not invade or metastasize. Researchers divide the causes of cancer into two groups: those with an environmental cause and those with a hereditary genetic cause.

Immunotherapy	Immunotherapy is a medical term defined as "treatment of disease by inducing, enhancing, or suppressing an immune response". Immunotherapies designed to elicit or amplify an immune response are classified as activation immunotherapies. Immunotherapies designed to reduce, suppress or more appropriately direct an existing immune response, as in cases of autoimmunity or allergy, are classified as suppression immunotherapies.
Pregnancy	Pregnancy is the carrying of one or more offspring, known as a fetus or embryo, inside the womb of a female. In a pregnancy, there can be multiple gestations, as in the case of twins or triplets. Human pregnancy is the most studied of all mammalian pregnancies.
Diabetes mellitus	Diabetes mellitus, often simply referred to as diabetes--is a group of metabolic diseases in which a person has high blood sugar, either because the body does not produce enough insulin, or because cells do not respond to the insulin that is produced. This high blood sugar produces the classical symptoms of polyuria (frequent urination), polydipsia (increased thirst) and polyphagia (increased hunger). There are three main types of diabetes: • Type 1 diabetes: results from the body's failure to produce insulin, and presently requires the person to inject insulin.
Atresia	Atresia is a condition in which a body orifice or passage in the body is abnormally closed or absent.

Examples of atresia include:

- Imperforate anus - malformation of the opening between the rectum and anus.
- Microtia- Absence of the ear canal or failure of the canal to be tubular or fully formed (can be related to Microtia- a congenital deformity of the pinna (outer ear)).
- Biliary atresia - Condition in newborns in which the common bile duct between the liver and the small intestine is blocked or absent.
- Choanal atresia - blockage of the back of the nasal passage, usually by abnormal bony or soft tissue.
- Esophageal atresia - affects the alimentary tract causing the esophagus to end before connecting normally to the stomach.
- Intestinal atresia - malformation of the intestine, usually resulting from a vascular accident in utero
- Ovarian follicle atresia, atresia refers to the degeneration and subsequent resorption of one or more immature ovarian follicles.
- Pulmonary atresia - malformation of the pulmonary valve in which the valve orifice fails to develop.
- Tricuspid atresia - a form of congenital heart disease whereby there is a complete absence of the tricuspid valve. Therefore, there is an absence of right atrioventricular connection.
- Vaginal atresia - congenital occlusion of the vagina or subsequence adhesion of the walls of the vagina occluding it.
- Potter sequence - congenital decreased size of the kidney leading absolute no functionality of the kidney, usually related to a single kidney.
- Aural Atresia - refers to the absence of an external ear canal, often with malformation of the external, middle, and/or inner ear.

Ureterocele

A ureterocele is a congenital abnormality found in the urinary bladder. In this condition called ureteroceles, the distal ureter balloons at its opening into the bladder, forming a sac-like pouch. It is most often associated with a duplicated collection system, where two ureters drain their respective kidney instead of one.

Megaureter

Megaureter is an anomaly whereby the ureter is abnormally dilated. Congenital megaureter is an uncommon condition which is more common in males, may be bilateral, and is often associated with other congenital anomalies. The cause is thought to be aperistalsis of the distal ureter, leading to dilatation.

Percutaneous	In surgery, percutaneous pertains to any medical procedure where access to inner organs or other tissue is done via needle-puncture of the skin, rather than by using an "open" approach where inner organs or tissue are exposed (typically with the use of a scalpel). The percutaneous approach is commonly used in vascular procedures. This involves a needle catheter getting access to a blood vessel, followed by the introduction of a wire through the lumen (pathway) of the needle.
Retroperitoneal fibrosis	Retroperitoneal fibrosis is a disease featuring the proliferation of fibrous tissue in the retroperitoneum, the compartment of the body containing the kidneys, aorta, renal tract and various other structures. It may present with lower back pain, renal failure, hypertension, deep vein thrombosis and other obstructive symptoms. It is named after John Kelso Ormond, who rediscovered the condition in 1948.
Interstitial cystitis	Interstitial cystitis is a chronic, severely debilitating disease of the urinary bladder. Of unknown cause, it is characterised by: pain associated with the bladder, pain associated with urination (dysuria), urinary frequency (as often as every 10 minutes), urgency, and/or pressure in the bladder and/or pelvis. The disease has a profound impact on quality of life.
Pathogenesis	The term pathogenesis means step by step development of a disease and the chain of events leading to that disease due to a series of changes in the structure and/or function of a cell/tissue/organ being caused by a microbial, chemical or physical agent. The pathogenesis of a disease is the mechanism by which a disease is caused. The term can also be used to describe the development of the disease, such as acute, chronic and recurrent.
Schistosomiasis	Schistosomiasis is a parasitic disease caused by several species of trematodes (platyhelminth infection, or "flukes"), a parasitic worm of the genus Schistosoma.

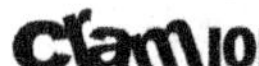

Although it has a low mortality rate, schistosomiasis often is a chronic illness that can damage internal organs and, in children, impair growth and cognitive development. The urinary form of schistosomiasis is associated with increased risks for bladder cancer in adults.

Enuresis

Enuresis refers to an inability to control urination. Use of the term is usually limited to describing individuals old enough to be expected to exercise such control.

Types of enuresis include:

- Nocturnal enuresis
- Diurnal enuresis

The controversial diagnosis PANDAS (pediatric autoimmune neuropsychiatric disorders associated with streptococcal infections) has been used to describe a set of children who have a rapid onset of OCD and/or tic disorders following a streptococcal infection, with a link to other symptoms such as enuresis.

Prolapse

Prolapse literally means "to fall out of place". In medicine, prolapse is a condition where organs, such as the uterus, fall down or slip out of place. It is used for organs protruding through the vagina or the rectum or for the misalignment of the valves of the heart.

Psychodynamics

Psychodynamics is the theory and systematic study of the psychological forces that underlie human behavior, especially the dynamic relations between conscious motivation and unconscious motivation. The psychologist Sigmund Freud (1856-1939) developed "psychodynamics" to describe the processes of the mind as flows of psychological energy (Libido) in an organically complex brain.

In medical praxis, psychodynamic psychotherapy is a less intensive, 3-5 weekly sessions, than the classical Freudian psychoanalysis treatment of only one weekly session.

Urethra	In anatomy, the urethra is a tube that connects the urinary bladder to the genitals for removal out of the body. In males, the urethra travels through the penis, and carries semen as well as urine. In females, the urethra is shorter and emerges above the vaginal opening.
Lipoma	A lipoma is a benign tumor composed of adipose tissue. It is the most common form of soft tissue tumor. Lipomas are soft to the touch, usually movable, and are generally painless.
Radiation	In physics, radiation describes a process in which energetic particles or waves travel through a medium or space. There are two distinct types of radiation; ionizing and non-ionizing. The word radiation is commonly used in reference to ionizing radiation only (i.e., having sufficient energy to ionize an atom), but it may also refer to non-ionizing radiation.
Diethylstilbestrol	Diethylstilbestrol is a synthetic nonsteroidal estrogen that was first synthesized in 1938. Human exposure to DES occurred through diverse sources, such as dietary ingestion from supplemented cattle feed and medical treatment for certain conditions, including breast and prostate cancers. From about 1940 to 1970, DES was given to pregnant women under the mistaken belief it would reduce the risk of pregnancy complications and losses. In 1971, DES was shown to cause a rare vaginal tumor in girls and young women who had been exposed to this drug in utero.
Ejaculation	Ejaculation is the ejecting of semen (usually carrying sperm) from the male reproductory tract, and is usually accompanied by orgasm. It is usually the final stage and natural objective of sexual stimulation, and an essential component of natural conception. In rare cases ejaculation occurs because of prostatic disease.
Seminal vesicle	The seminal vesicles (glandulae vesiculosae) or vesicular glands are a pair of simple tubular glands posteroinferior to the urinary bladder of male mammals. Anatomy Each seminal gland spreads approximately 5 cm, though the full length of seminal vesicle is approximately 10 cm, but it is curled up inside of the gland's structure. Each gland forms as an outpocketing of the wall of ampulla of each vas deferens.

Priapism	Priapism, known also as Hulseyism, is a potentially harmful and painful medical condition in which the erect penis or clitoris does not return to its flaccid state, despite the absence of both physical and psychological stimulation, within four hours. There are two types of priapism: low-flow and high-flow. Low-flow involves the blood not adequately returning to the body from the organ.
Sertoli cell	A Sertoli cell is a 'nurse' cell of the testes that is part of a seminiferous tubule. It is activated by follicle-stimulating hormone and has FSH-receptor on its membranes. Functions Because its main function is to nurture the developing sperm cells through the stages of spermatogenesis, the Sertoli cell has also been called the "mother" or "nurse" cell.
Hormone	A hormone is a chemical released by a cell or a gland in one part of the body that sends out messages that affect cells in other parts of the organism. Only a small amount of hormone is required to alter cell metabolism. In essence, it is a chemical messenger that transports a signal from one cell to another.
Sexual function	Sexual function is a model developed at the Karolinska Institute in Stockholm, Sweden, defining different aspects of the assessment of sexual dysfunction comprises the following components. Firstly, relevant aspects of sexual function are defined on the basis of a modified version of Masters and Johnson's pioneer work. The aspects of sexual function defined as being relevant to the assessment include sexual desire, erection, orgasm and ejaculation.
Pharmacology	Pharmacology is the branch of medicine and biology concerned with the study of drug action. More specifically, it is the study of the interactions that occur between a living organism and chemicals that affect normal or abnormal biochemical function. If substances have medicinal properties, they are considered pharmaceuticals.

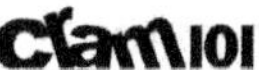

Premature ejaculation	Premature ejaculation is a condition in which a man ejaculates earlier than he or his partner would like him to. Premature ejaculation is also known as rapid ejaculation, rapid climax, premature climax, or early ejaculation. Masters and Johnson defines Premature ejaculation as the condition in which a man ejaculates before his sex partner achieves orgasm, in more than fifty percent of their sexual encounters.
Retrograde ejaculation	In the human male reproductive system, retrograde ejaculation occurs when semen, which would normally be ejaculated via the urethra, is redirected to the urinary bladder. Normally, the sphincter of the bladder contracts before ejaculation forcing the semen to exit via the urethra, the path of least pressure. When the bladder sphincter does not function properly, retrograde ejaculation may occur.
Epidemiology	Epidemiology is the study of patterns of health and illness and associated factors at the population level. It is the cornerstone method of public health research, and helps inform evidence-based medicine for identifying risk factors for disease and determining optimal treatment approaches to clinical practice and for preventative medicine. In the study of communicable and non-communicable diseases, epidemiologists are involved in outbreak investigation to study design, data collection, statistical analysis, documentation of results and submission for publication.
Androgen	Androgen, is the generic term for any natural or synthetic compound, usually a steroid hormone, that stimulates or controls the development and maintenance of male characteristics in vertebrates by binding to androgen receptors. This includes the activity of the accessory male sex organs and development of male secondary sex characteristics. Androgens were first discovered in 1936. Androgens are also the original anabolic steroids and the precursor of all estrogens, the female sex hormones.
Penicillin	Penicillin is a group of antibiotics derived from Penicillium fungi. Penicillin antibiotics are historically significant because they are the first drugs that were effective against many previously serious diseases such as syphilis and Staphylococcus infections. Penicillins are still widely used today, though many types of bacteria are now resistant.
Prostatitis	Prostatitis is an inflammation of the prostate gland, in men. A prostatitis diagnosis is assigned at 8% of all urologist and 1% of all primary care physician visits in the United States. Classification

	The term prostatitis refers, in its strictest sense, to histological (microscopic) inflammation of the tissue of the prostate gland.
Syphilis	Syphilis is a sexually transmitted disease caused by the spirochetal bacteria Treponema pallidum subspecies pallidum. The primary route of transmission of syphilis is through sexual contact however it may also be transmitted from mother to fetus during pregnancy or at birth resulting in congenital syphilis. The signs and symptoms of syphilis vary depending on which of the four stages it presents in (primary, secondary, latent, and tertiary).
Systemic disease	Life-threatening disease redirects here. A systemic disease is one that affects a number of organs and tissues, or affects the body as a whole. Although most medical conditions will eventually involve multiple organs in advanced stage (e.g. Multiple organ dysfunction syndrome), diseases where multiple organ involvement is at presentation or in early stage are considered elsewhere.
Intracavernous injection	An intracavernous (or intracavernosal) injection is an injection into the base of the penis. This injection site is often used to administer medications to check for or treat erectile dysfunction in adult men (in e.g. combined intracavernous injection and stimulation test).

Duplex ultrasonography	Duplex ultrasonography is a form of medical ultrasonography that incorporates two elements: • 1) Grayscale Ultrasound to visualize the structure or architecture of the body part. No motion or bloodflow is assessed. This is the way plaque is directly imaged in a blood vessel, with the reader typically commenting on crossectional narrowing (greater than 70% is typically considered worthy of treatment). • 2) Color-doppler Ultrasound to visualize the flow or movement of a structure, typically used to image blood within an artery.
Nocturnal penile tumescence	Nocturnal penile tumescence is the spontaneous occurrence of an erection of the penis during sleep. Most men without physiological erectile dysfunction experience this phenomenon, usually three to five times during the night. It typically happens during REM sleep.
Tumescence	Tumescence is the quality or state of being tumescent or swollen. This swelling includes expanding foam and expanding caulk. Tumescence usually refers to the normal engorgement with blood (vascular congestion) of the erectile tissues, marking sexual excitation and possible readiness for sexual activity.
Phosphodiesterase inhibitor	A phosphodiesterase inhibitor is a drug that blocks one or more of the five subtypes of the enzyme phosphodiesterase (PDE), therefore preventing the inactivation of the intracellular second messengers cyclic adenosine monophosphate (cAMP) and cyclic guanosine monophosphate (cGMP) by the respective PDE subtype(s). History The different forms or subtypes of phosphodiesterase were initially isolated from rat brains by Uzunov and Weiss in 1972 and were soon afterwards shown to be selectively inhibited in the brain and in other tissues by a variety of drugs. The potential for selective phosphodiesterase inhibitors as therapeutic agents was predicted as early as 1977 by Weiss and Hait.

Prostate-specific antigen	Prostate-specific antigen is a protein produced by the cells of the prostate gland. Prostate specific antigen is present in small quantities in the serum of men with healthy prostates, but is often elevated in the presence of prostate cancer and in other prostate disorders. A blood test to measure Prostate specific antigen is considered the most effective test currently available for the early detection of prostate cancer, but this effectiveness has also been questioned.
Sildenafil	Sildenafil citrate, sold as Viagra, Revatio and under various other trade names, is a drug used to treat erectile dysfunction and pulmonary arterial hypertension (PAH). It was developed and is being marketed by the pharmaceutical company Pfizer. It acts by inhibiting cGMP-specific phosphodiesterase type 5, an enzyme that regulates blood flow in the penis.
Tadalafil	Tadalafil is a PDE5 inhibitor, currently marketed in pill form for treating erectile dysfunction (ED) under the name Cialis; and under the name Adcirca for the treatment of pulmonary arterial hypertension. It initially was developed by the biotechnology company ICOS, and then again developed and marketed world-wide by Lilly ICOS, LLC, the joint venture of ICOS Corporation and Eli Lilly and Company. Cialis tablets, in 5 mg, 10 mg, and 20 mg doses, are yellow, film-coated, and almond-shaped.
Vardenafil	Vardenafil is a PDE5 inhibitor used for treating impotence (erectile dysfunction) that is sold under the trade name Levitra (Bayer AG, GSK, and SP). History Vardenafil was co-marketed by Bayer Pharmaceuticals, GSK, and SP under the trade name Levitra. As of 2005, the co-promotion rights of GSK on Levitra have been returned to Bayer in many markets outside the U.S. In Italy, Bayer sells vardenafil as Levitra and GSK sells it as Vivanza, thus, because of European Union trade rules, parallel imports might result in Vivanza sold next to Levitra in the EU. Clinical use Vardenafil's indications and contra-indications are the same as with other PDE5 inhibitors; it is closely related in function to sildenafil citrate (Viagra) and tadalafil (Cialis).

Antigen	An antigen is a substance/molecule that, when introduced into the body, triggers the production of an antibody by the immune system, which will then kill or neutralize the antigen that is recognized as a foreign and potentially harmful invader. These invaders can be molecules such as pollen or cells such as bacteria. The term originally came from antibody generator and was a molecule that binds specifically to an antibody, but the term now also refers to any molecule or molecular fragment that can be bound by a major histocompatibility complex (MHC) and presented to a T-cell receptor.
Mechanism of action	In pharmacology, the term mechanism of action refers to the specific biochemical interaction through which a drug substance produces its pharmacological effect. A mechanism of action usually includes mention of the specific molecular targets to which the drug binds, such as an enzyme or receptor. For example, the mechanism of action of aspirin involves irreversible inhibition of the enzyme cyclooxygenase, which suppresses the production of prostaglandins and thromboxanes, thereby reducing pain and inflammation.
Testosterone	Testosterone is a steroid hormone from the androgen group and is found in mammals, reptiles, birds, and other vertebrates. In mammals, testosterone is primarily secreted in the testes of males and the ovaries of females, although small amounts are also secreted by the adrenal glands. It is the principal male sex hormone and an anabolic steroid.
Adverse event	An adverse event is any adverse change in health or side effect that occurs in a person who participates in a clinical trial while the patient is receiving the treatment (study medication, application of the study device, etc). or within a previously specified period of time after the treatment has been completed. Adverse events in patients participating in clinical trials must be reported to the local institutional review board (IRB) and the study sponsor.

Apomorphine

Apomorphine is a non-selective dopamine agonist which activates both D_1-like and D_2-like receptors, with some preference for the latter subtypes. It is historically a morphine decomposition product by boiling with concentrated acid, hence the -morphine suffix. Apomorphine does not actually contain morphine or its skeleton, or bind to opioid receptors for that matter.

Radiology

Radiology is medical specialty that employs the use of imaging to both diagnose and treat disease visualized within the human body. Radiologists utilize an array of imaging technologies (such as x-ray radiography, ultrasound, computed tomography (CT), nuclear medicine, positron emission tomography (PET) and magnetic resonance imaging (MRI)) to diagnose or treat diseases. Interventional radiology is the performance of (usually minimally invasive) medical procedures with the guidance of imaging technologies.

Papaverine

Papaverine is an opium alkaloid used primarily in the treatment of visceral spasm, vasospasm (especially those involving the heart and the brain), and occasionally in the treatment of erectile dysfunction. While it is found in the opium poppy, papaverine differs in both structure and pharmacological action from the analgesic (morphine-related) opium alkaloids (opioids).

Uses

Papaverine is approved to treat spasms of the gastrointestinal tract, bile ducts and ureter and for use as a cerebral and coronary vasodilator in subarachnoid hemorrhage (combined with balloon angioplasty) and coronary artery bypass surgery. Papaverine may also be used as a smooth muscle relaxant in microsurgery where it is applied directly to blood vessels.

Papaverine is used as an erectile dysfunction drug, alone or sometimes in combination.

Adverse effect

In medicine, an adverse effect is a harmful and undesired effect resulting from a medication or other intervention such as surgery. An adverse effect may be termed a "side effect", when judged to be secondary to a main or therapeutic effect. If it results from an unsuitable or incorrect dosage or procedure, this is called a medical error and not a complication.

Contraindication

In medicine, a contraindication is a condition or factor that serves as a reason to withhold a certain medical treatment.

	Some contraindications are absolute, meaning that there are no reasonable circumstances for undertaking a course of action. For example, children and teenagers with viral infections should not be given aspirin because of the risk of Reye's syndrome, and a person with an anaphylactic food allergy should never eat the food to which they are allergic.
Surgery	Surgery is an ancient medical specialty that uses operative manual and instrumental techniques on a patient to investigate and/or treat a pathological condition such as disease or injury, to help improve bodily function or appearance, and sometimes for religious reasons. An act of performing surgery may be called a surgical procedure, operation, or simply surgery. In this context, the verb operate means performing surgery.
Penile prosthesis	A penile prosthesis is a medical device implanted in the penis requiring a surgical procedure. The device is often used for men with organic or treatment-resistant psychogenic impotence who suffer from erectile dysfunction. A penile prosthesis is also used in the final stage of plastic surgery phalloplasty to complete female to male gender reassignment surgery as well as during total phalloplasty for adult and child patients that need male genital modification.
Physiology	Physiology is the science of the function of living systems. It is a subcategory of biology. In physiology, the scientific method is applied to determine how organisms, organ systems, organs, cells and biomolecules carry out the chemical or physical function that they have in a living system.
Enterocele	Enterocele is a protrusion of the small intestines and peritoneum into the vaginal canal. It can be treated transvaginally or by laparoscopy.
Sexual dysfunction	Sexual dysfunction, including desire, arousal or orgasm.

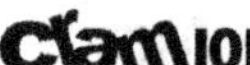

	To maximize the benefits of medications and behavioural techniques in the management of sexual dysfunction it is important to have a comprehensive approach to the problem,A thorough sexual history and assessment of general health and other sexual problems (if any) are very important. Assessing (performance) anxiety, guilt (associated with masturbation in many South-Asian men), stress and worry are integral to the optimal management of sexual dysfunction.
Micropenis	Micropenis is an unusually small penis. A common criterion is a dorsal (measured on top) erect penile length of at least 2.5 standard deviations smaller than the mean human penis size. The condition is usually recognized shortly after birth.
Posterior urethral valve	Posterior urethral valve disorder is an obstructive developmental anomaly in the urethra and genitourinary system of male newborns. A posterior urethral valve is an obstructing membrane in the posterior male urethra as a result of abnormal in utero development. It is the most common cause of bladder outlet obstruction in male newborns.
Chordee	Chordee is a condition in which the head of the penis curves downward (that is, in a ventral direction) or upward, at the junction of the head and shaft of the penis. The curvature is usually most obvious during erection, but resistance to straightening is often apparent in the flaccid state as well. In many cases but not all, chordee is associated with hypospadias.
Hypospadias	Hypospadias is a birth defect of the urethra in the male that involves an abnormally placed urinary meatus (the opening, or male external urethral orifice). Instead of opening at the tip of the glans of the penis, a hypospadic urethra opens anywhere along a line (the urethral groove) running from the tip along the underside (ventral aspect) of the shaft to the junction of the penis and scrotum or perineum. A distal hypospadias may be suspected even in an uncircumcised boy from an abnormally formed foreskin and downward tilt of the glans.
Epispadias	An epispadias is a rare type of malformation of the penis in which the urethra ends in an opening on the upper aspect (the dorsum) of the penis. It can also develop in females when the urethra develops too far anteriorly. It occurs in around 1 in 120,000 male and 1 in 500,000 female births.
Circumcision	Male circumcision is the removal of some or all of the foreskin (prepuce) from the penis. The word "circumcision" comes from Latin circum (meaning "around") and cædere (meaning "to cut"). Early depictions of circumcision are found in cave paintings and Ancient Egyptian tombs, though some pictures are open to interpretation.

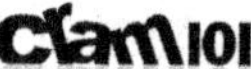

Paraphimosis	Paraphimosis is an uncommon medical condition where the foreskin becomes trapped behind the glans penis, and cannot be reduced (that is, pulled back to its normal flaccid position covering the glans penis). If this condition persists for several hours or there is any sign of a lack of blood flow, paraphimosis should be treated as a medical emergency, as it can result in gangrene or other serious complications. Paraphimosis is usually caused by well-meaning medical professionals or parents who handle the foreskin improperly: The foreskin may be retracted during penile examination, penile cleaning, urethral catheterization, or cystoscopy; if the foreskin is left retracted for a long period of time, some of the foreskin tissue may become edematous (swollen with fluid), which makes subsequent reduction of the foreskin difficult.
Penis	The penis is a biological feature of male animals including both vertebrates and invertebrates. It is a reproductive, intromittent organ that additionally serves as the urinal duct in placental mammals. Etymology The word "penis" is taken from the Latin word for "tail." Some derive that from Indo-European *pesnis, and the Greek word π?ος = "penis" from Indo-European *pesos.
Phimosis	Phimosis is a condition where, in men, the male foreskin cannot be fully retracted from the head of the penis. The term may also refer to clitoral phimosis in women, whereby the clitoral hood cannot be retracted, limiting exposure of the glans clitoridis. In the neonatal period, it is rare for the foreskin to be retractable; Huntley et al. state that "non-retractability can be considered normal for males up to and including adolescence." Rickwood, as well as other authors, has suggested that true phimosis is over-diagnosed due to failure to distinguish between normal developmental non-retractability and a pathological condition (a condition deemed a problem).

Urethrotomy	A urethrotomy is an operation which involves incision of the urethra, especially for relief of a stricture. Direct visual internal urethrotomy uses an endoscopic device known as a urethrotome. This is inserted up the urethra to the stricture and an extendible knife (or laser) is used to make the incisions.
Meatal stenosis	Urethral meatal stenosis is a narrowing (stenosis) of the opening of the urethra at the external meatus, thus constricting the opening through which urine leaves the body from the urinary bladder. Causes, incidence, and risk factors Studies have indicated that male circumcision contributes to the development of urethral stricture. Among circumcised males, reported incidence figures include 0%, 0.01%, 0.55%, 0.9%, 2.8%, 7.29%, 9-10%, and 11%.
Stenosis	A stenosis is an abnormal narrowing in a blood vessel or other tubular organ or structure. It is also sometimes called a stricture (as in urethral stricture). The term coarctation is synonymous, but is commonly used only in the context of aortic coarctation.
Ureaplasma urealyticum	Ureaplasma urealyticum is a bacterium belonging to the family Mycoplasmataceae. Its type strain is T960. Clinical significance

	U. urealyticum is part of the normal genital flora of both men and women.
Diverticulum	A diverticulum is medical or biological term for an outpouching of a hollow (or a fluid filled) structure in the body. In medicine the term usually implies that the structure is not normally present, i.e., pathological. However, in the embryonic stage, some normal structures begin development as a diverticulum arising from another structure.
Contact dermatitis	Contact dermatitis is a term for a skin reaction (dermatitis) resulting from exposure to allergens (allergic contact dermatitis) or irritants (irritant contact dermatitis). Phototoxic dermatitis occurs when the allergen or irritant is activated by sunlight. Symptoms Contact dermatitis is a localized rash or irritation of the skin caused by contact with a foreign substance.
Intertrigo	An intertrigo is an inflammation (rash) of the body folds (adjacent areas of skin). An intertrigo sometimes refers to a bacterial, fungal, or viral infection that has developed at the site of broken skin due to such inflammation. A frequent manifestation is Candidal intertrigo.
Lichen simplex chronicus	Lichen simplex chronicus is a skin disorder characterized by chronic itching and scratching. The constant scratching causes thick, leathery, brownish skin.

This is a skin disorder characterized by a self-perpetuating scratch-itch cycle:

- It may begin with something that rubs, irritates, or scratches the skin, such as clothing.
- This causes the person to rub or scratch the affected area.

Psoriasis

Psoriasis is a chronic autoimmune disease that appears on the skin. It occurs when the immune system sends out faulty signals that speed up the growth cycle of skin cells. Psoriasis is not contagious.

Candidiasis

Candidiasis is a fungal infection (mycosis) of any of the Candida species (all yeasts), of which Candida albicans is the most common. Also commonly referred to as a yeast infection, candidiasis is also technically known as candidosis, moniliasis, and oidiomycosis.

Candidiasis encompasses infections that range from superficial, such as oral thrush and vaginitis, to systemic and potentially life-threatening diseases.

Drug eruption

In medicine, a drug eruption is an adverse drug reaction of the skin. Most drug-induced cutaneous reactions are mild and disappear when the offending drug is withdrawn. Drugs can also cause hair and nail changes, affect the mucous membranes, or cause itching without outward skin changes.

Crab

True crabs are decapod crustaceans of the infraorder Brachyura, which typically have a very short projecting "tail", or where the reduced abdomen is entirely hidden under the thorax. Many other animals with similar names - such as hermit crabs, king crabs, porcelain crabs, horseshoe crabs and crab lice - are not true crabs.

Evolution

Crabs are generally covered with a thick exoskeleton, and armed with a single pair of chelae (claws).

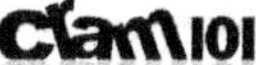

Lichen planus	Lichen planus is a chronic mucocutaneous disease that affects the skin, tongue, and oral mucosa. The disease presents itself in the form of papules, lesions, or rashes. Lichen planus does not involve lichens; the name refers to the appearance of affected skin.
Lichen sclerosus	Lichen sclerosus (also known as "Lichen sclerosus et atrophicus") is an uncommon disease of unknown cause that results in white patches on the skin, which may cause scarring on and around genital skin. Several risk factors have been proposed, including autoimmune diseases, infections and genetic predisposition. There is evidence that lichen sclerosus can be associated with thyroid disease..
Pediculosis	Pediculosis is an infestation of lice -- blood-feeding ectoparasitic insects of the order Phthiraptera. The condition can occur in almost any species of warm-blooded animal (i.e., mammals and birds), including humans. Although "pediculosis" in humans may properly refer to lice infestation of any part of the body, the term is sometimes used loosely to refer to pediculosis capitis, the infestation of the human head with the specific head louse.
Pediculosis pubis	Pediculosis pubis is a disease caused by the crab louse Phthirus pubis, a parasitic insect notorious for infesting human genitals. The species may also live on other areas with hair, including the eyelashes causing pediculosis ciliaris. Infestation usually lead to intense itching in the pubic area.
Scabies	Scabies, known colloquial as the seven-year itch, is a contagious skin infection that occurs among humans and other animals. It is caused by a tiny and usually not directly visible parasite, the mite Sarcoptes scabiei, which burrows under the host's skin, causing intense allergic itching. The word scabies is derived from the Latin word scabere, to scratch.
Tinea cruris	Tinea cruris, crotch rot, eczema marginatum, gym itch, jock itch, and ringworm of the groin in American English is a dermatophyte fungal infection of the groin region in either sex, though more often seen in males. Symptoms and signs

As the common name for this condition implies, it causes itching or a burning sensation in the groin area, thigh skin folds, or anus. It may involve the inner thighs and genital areas, as well as extending back to the perineum and perianal areas.

Cephalosporin

The cephalosporins are a class of β-lactam antibiotics originally derived from Acremonium, which was previously known as "Cephalosporium".

Together with cephamycins they constitute a subgroup of β-lactam antibiotics called cephems.

History

Cephalosporin compounds were first isolated from cultures of Cephalosporium acremonium from a sewer in Sardinia in 1948 by Italian scientist Giuseppe Brotzu.

Folliculitis

Folliculitis is the inflammation of one or more hair follicles. The condition may occur anywhere on the skin.

Most carbuncles, furuncles, and other cases of folliculitis develop from Staphylococcus aureus.

Molluscum contagiosum

Molluscum contagiosum is a viral infection of the skin or occasionally of the mucous membranes. It is caused by a DNA poxvirus called the molluscum contagiosum virus (MCV). MCV has no animal reservoir, infecting only humans.

Genital wart

Genital warts (or Condylomata acuminata, venereal warts, anal warts and anogenital warts) is a highly contagious sexually transmitted disease caused by some sub-types of human papillomavirus (HPV). It is spread through direct skin-to-skin contact during oral, genital, or anal sex with an infected partner. Warts are the most easily recognized symptom of genital HPV infection, where types 6 and 11 are responsible for 90% of genital warts cases.

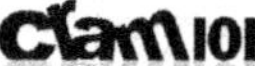

Wart	A wart is generally a small, rough growth, typically on hands and feet but often other locations, that can resemble a cauliflower or a solid blister. They are caused by a viral infection, specifically by human papillomavirus 2 and 7. There are as many as 10 varieties of warts with the most common being considered largely harmless. It is possible to get warts from others; they are contagious.
Herpes simplex	Herpes simplex is a viral disease caused by both herpes simplex virus type 1 (HSV-1) and type 2 (HSV-2). Infection with the herpes virus is categorized into one of several distinct disorders based on the site of infection. Oral herpes, the visible symptoms of which are colloquially called cold sores or fever blisters, infects the face and mouth.
Herpes simplex virus	Herpes simplex virus 1 and 2 (Herpes simplex virus-1 and Herpes simplex virus-2), also known as Human herpes virus 1 and 2 (HHV-1 and -2), are two members of the herpes virus family, Herpesviridae, that infect humans. Both Herpes simplex virus-1 (which produces cold sores) and Herpes simplex virus-2 (which produces genital herpes) are ubiquitous and contagious. They can be spread when an infected person is producing and shedding the virus.
Sex assignment	Sex assignment refers to the assigning of sex at the birth of a baby. In the majority of births, a relative, midwife, or physician inspects the genitalia when the baby is delivered, sees ordinary male or female genitalia, and declares, "it's a girl" or "it's a boy" without hesitation or uncertainty. The assignment is perceived as a recognition of an essential aspect of this new human being, apparent to everyone.
Rectocele	A rectocele results from a tear in the rectovaginal septum (which is normally a tough, fibrous, sheet-like divider between the rectum and vagina). Rectal tissue bulges through this tear and into the vagina as a hernia. There are two main causes of this tear: childbirth, and hysterectomy.
Turner syndrome	Turner syndrome, of which monosomy X (absence of an entire sex chromosome, the Barr body) is most common. It is a chromosomal abnormality in which all or part of one of the sex chromosomes is absent (unaffected humans have 46 chromosomes, of which two are sex chromosomes). Typical females have two X chromosomes, but in Turner syndrome, one of those sex chromosomes is missing or has other abnormalities.
True hermaphroditism	True hermaphroditism is a medical term for an intersex condition in which an individual is born with ovarian and testicular tissue.

	There may be an ovary on one side and a testis on the other, but more commonly one or both gonads is an ovotestis containing both types of tissue. It is rare--so far undocumented--for both types of gonadal tissue to function.
Cloacal exstrophy	Cloacal exstrophy is a severe birth defect wherein much of the abdominal organs (the bladder and intestines) are exposed. It often causes the splitting of both male and female genitalia (specifically, the penis and clitoris respectively), and the anus is occasionally sealed. Cloacal exstrophy is an extremely rare birth defect, present in only one in 250,000 births.
Clitoroplasty	Clitoroplasty is a term for the surgical creation (in trans women as part of gender reassignment surgery) of a clitoris, or restoration, in the case of a procedure to reverse the damage caused by female genital multilation. People with congenital adrenal hyperplasia may also undergo this to correct genital anatomy or complications of the condition. It is rarely performed on ciswomen for cosmetic reasons.
Vaginoplasty	Vaginoplasty is a reconstructive surgery procedure used to either construct or reconstruct a vaginal canal and its mucous membrane. As such, the term vaginoplasty generally describes any such vaginal surgery, and the term neovaginoplasty specifically describes the procedures of either partial or total construction, or reconstruction, of the vulvovaginal complex. These bodily structures might be absent from a woman, because of congenital disease (e.g. vaginal atresia) or because of an acquired cause (e.g. physical trauma, cancer).

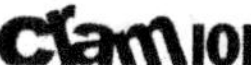

Hypothalamus	The Hypothalamus is a portion of the brain that contains a number of small nuclei with a variety of functions. One of the most important functions of the hypothalamus is to link the nervous system to the endocrine system via the pituitary gland (hypophysis). The hypothalamus is located below the thalamus, just above the brain stem.
Feedback	Feedback describes the situation when output from (or information about the result of) an event or phenomenon in the past will influence an occurrence or occurrences of the same (i.e. same defined) event / phenomenon (or the continuation / development of the original phenomenon) in the present or future. When an event is part of a chain of cause-and-effect that forms a circuit or loop, then the event is said to "feed back" into itself. Feedback is also a synonym for: • Feedback signal - the information about the initial event that is the basis for subsequent modification of the event • Feedback loop - the causal path that leads from the initial generation of the feedback signal to the subsequent modification of the event • Audio feedback - the special kind of positive feedback that occurs when a loop exists between an audio input and output. Overview Feedback is a mechanism, process or signal that is looped back to control a system within itself.
Anterior pituitary	A major organ of the endocrine system, the anterior pituitary, is the glandular, anterior lobe of the pituitary gland. The anterior pituitary regulates several physiological processes including stress, growth, and reproduction.

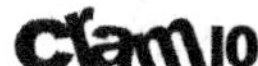

Its regulatory functions are achieved through the secretion of various peptide hormones that act on target organs including the adrenal gland, liver, bone, thyroid gland, and gonads.

Follicle-stimulating hormone

Follicle-stimulating hormone is a hormone found in humans and other animals. It is synthesized and secreted by gonadotrophs of the anterior pituitary gland. Follicle stimulating hormone regulates the development, growth, pubertal maturation, and reproductive processes of the body.

Male infertility

Male infertility refers to the inability of a male to achieve a pregnancy in a fertile female. In humans it accounts for 40-50% of infertility. Male infertility is commonly due to deficiencies in the semen, and semen quality is used as a surrogate measure of male fecundity.

Spermatogenesis

Spermatogenesis is the process by which male primary germ cells undergo division, and produce a number of cells termed spermatogonia, from which the primary spermatocytes are derived. Each primary spermatocyte divides into two secondary spermatocytes, and each secondary spermatocyte into two spermatids or young spermatozoa. These develop into mature spermatozoa, also known as sperm cells.

Germ cell

A germ cell is any biological cell that gives rise to the gametes of an organism that reproduces sexually. In many animals, the germ cells originate near the gut of an embryo and migrate to the developing gonads. There, they undergo cell division of two types, mitosis and meiosis, followed by cellular differentiation into mature gametes, either eggs or sperm.

Sperm

The term sperm is derived from the Greek word (σπ?ρμα) sperma and refers to the male reproductive cells. In the types of sexual reproduction known as anisogamy and oogamy, there is a marked difference in the size of the gametes with the smaller one being termed the "male" or sperm cell. The human sperm cell is haploid, so that its 23 chromosomes can join the 23 chromosomes of the female egg to form a diploid cell.

Y chromosome

The Y chromosome is one of the two sex-determining chromosomes in most mammals, including humans. In mammals, it contains the gene SRY, which triggers testis development if present. The human Y chromosome is composed of about 60 million base pairs.

Epididymis	The epididymis is part of the male reproductive system and is present in all male amniotes. It is a narrow, tightly-coiled tube connecting the efferent ducts from the rear of each testicle to its vas deferens. A similar, but probably non-homologous, structure is found in cartilaginous fishes.
Cryptorchidism	Cryptorchidism is the absence of one or both testes from the scrotum. It is the most common birth defect regarding male genitalia. In unique cases, cryptorchidism can develop later in life, often as late as young adulthood.
Orchidometer	An orchidometer is a medical instrument used to measure the volume of the testicles. The orchidometer was introduced in 1966 by pediatric endocrinologist Prof. Dr. Dr. hc.
Semen	Semen is an organic fluid, also known as seminal fluid, that may contain spermatozoa. It is secreted by the gonads (sexual glands) and other sexual organs of male or hermaphroditic animals and can fertilize female ova. In humans, seminal fluid contains several components besides spermatozoa: proteolytic and other enzymes as well as fructose are elements of seminal fluid which promote the survival of spermatozoa and provide a medium through which they can move or "swim".
Varicocele	Varicocele is an abnormal enlargement of the vein that is in the scrotum draining the testicles. The testicular blood vessels originate in the abdomen and course down through the inguinal canal as part of the spermatic cord on their way to the testis. Upward flow of blood in the veins is ensured by small one-way valves that prevent backflow.
Semen analysis	A semen analysis evaluates certain characteristics of a male's semen and the sperm contained in the semen. It may be done while investigating a couple's infertility or after a vasectomy to verify that the procedure was successful. It is also used for testing donors for sperm donation, in stud farming and farm animal breeding.
Urinalysis	A urinalysis is an array of tests performed on urine and one of the most common methods of medical diagnosis. A part of a urinalysis can be performed by using urine dipsticks, in which the test results can be read as color changes. Medical urinalysis

In addition to the substances mentioned in the table, other tests include:

- a description of color and appearance.
- Icotest - The test used to detect the destruction of old Red Blood Cells (RBC) in the urine.
- nitrites
- Hemoglobin Test - Hemolysis in the blood vessels, a rupture in the capillaries of the glomerulus, or hemorrhage in the urinary system may cause hemoglobin to appear in the urine.
- hCG - normally absent, this hormone appears in the urine of pregnant women.

Scrotum

In some male mammals the scrotum is a dual-chambered protuberance of skin and muscle containing the testicles and divided by a septum. It is an extension of the abdomen, and is located between the penis and anus. In humans and some other mammals, the base of the scrotum becomes covered with curly pubic hairs at puberty.

Venography

Venography is a procedure in which an x-ray of the veins, a venogram, is taken after a special dye is injected into the bone marrow or veins. The dye has to be injected constantly via a catheter. Therefore a venography is an invasive procedure.

Chemotherapy

Chemotherapy, in the most simple sense, is the treatment of an ailment by chemicals especially by killing micro-organisms or cancerous cells. In popular usage, it refers to antineoplastic drugs used to treat cancer or the combination of these drugs into a cytotoxic standardized treatment regimen. In its non-oncological use, the term may also refer to antibiotics (antibacterial chemotherapy).

Chromatin

Chromatin is the combination of DNA, histone, and other proteins that make up chromosomes. It is found inside the nuclear envelope of eukaryotic cells. It is divided between heterochromatin and euchromatin forms.

Mutation

In molecular biology and genetics, mutations are changes in a genomic sequence: the DNA sequence of a cell's genome or the DNA or RNA sequence of a virus. Mutations are caused by radiation, viruses, transposons and mutagenic chemicals, as well as errors that occur during meiosis or DNA replication. They can also be induced by the organism itself, by cellular processes such as hypermutation.

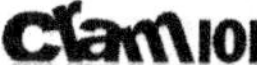

Kallmann syndrome	Kallmann syndrome is a hypogonadism (decreased functioning of the glands that produce sex hormones) caused by a deficiency of gonadotropin-releasing hormone (GnRH), which is created by the hypothalamus. Kallmann syndrome is also called hypothalamic hypogonadism, familial hypogonadism with anosmia, and hypogonadotropic hypogonadism, reflecting its disease mechanism. Kallmann syndrome is a form of tertiary hypogonadism, reflecting that the primary cause of the defect in sex-hormone production lies within the hypothalamus rather than a defect of the pituitary (secondary hypogonadism), testes or ovaries (primary hypogonadism).
Hypothalamic disease	A Hypothalamic disease is a disorder presenting primarily in the hypothalamus. An example is certain forms of neurogenic diabetes insipidus. Due to the tight integration of the hypothalamus and the pituitary, and the relative inaccessibility of these glands, it is often difficult to tell if a condition is due to dysfunction in the hypothalamus or in the pituitary, though certain hormone tests can help distinguish between these causes.
Cerebellar ataxia	Cerebellar ataxia is a form of ataxia originating in the cerebellum.
Estrogen	Estrogens (AmE), oestrogens (BE), or œstrogens, are a group of compounds named for their importance in the estrous cycle of humans and other animals, and functioning as the primary female sex hormones. Natural estrogens are steroid hormones, while some synthetic ones are non-steroidal. Their name comes from the Greek words estrus/ο?στρος = sexual desire + gen/γ?νο = to generate.
Pituitary disease	A Pituitary disease is a disorder primarily affecting the Pituitary gland. Disorders involving the pituitary gland include:

Androgen	Androgen, is the generic term for any natural or synthetic compound, usually a steroid hormone, that stimulates or controls the development and maintenance of male characteristics in vertebrates by binding to androgen receptors. This includes the activity of the accessory male sex organs and development of male secondary sex characteristics. Androgens were first discovered in 1936. Androgens are also the original anabolic steroids and the precursor of all estrogens, the female sex hormones.
Glucocorticoid	Glucocorticoids (GC) are a class of steroid hormones that bind to the glucocorticoid receptor (GR), which is present in almost every vertebrate animal cell. GCs are part of the feedback mechanism in the immune system that turns immune activity (inflammation) down. They are therefore used in medicine to treat diseases that are caused by an overactive immune system, such as allergies, asthma, autoimmune diseases and sepsis.
Growth hormone	Growth hormone is a protein-based peptide hormone. It stimulates growth, cell reproduction and regeneration in humans and other animals. Growth hormone is a 191-amino acid, single-chain polypeptide that is synthesized, stored, and secreted by the somatotroph cells within the lateral wings of the anterior pituitary gland.
Kidney transplantation	Kidney transplantation is the organ transplant of a kidney into a patient with end-stage renal disease. Kidney transplantation is typically classified as deceased-donor (formerly known as cadaveric) or living-donor transplantation depending on the source of the donor organ. Living-donor renal transplants are further characterized as genetically related (living-related) or non-related (living-unrelated) transplants, depending on whether a biological relationship exists between the donor and recipient.
XX male syndrome	XX male syndrome is a rare sex chromosomal disorder. Usually it is caused by unequal crossing over between X and Y chromosomes during meiosis, which results in one or both of the X chromosomes containing the normally-male SRY gene. This syndrome occurs in approximately four or five in 100,000 individuals, making it less common than Klinefelter syndrome.

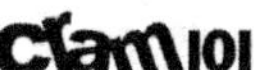

XYY syndrome	XYY syndrome is an aneuploidy (abnormal number) of the sex chromosomes in which a human male receives an extra Y chromosome, giving a total of 47 chromosomes instead of the more usual 46. This produces a 47,XYY karyotype. This condition is usually asymptomatic and affects 1 in 1000 male births. Some medical geneticists question whether the term "syndrome" is appropriate for this condition because its phenotype is normal and the vast majority (an estimated 97% in the UK) of 47,XYY males do not know their karyotype.
Myotonic dystrophy	Myotonic dystrophy is a chronic, slowly progressing, highly variable inherited multisystemic disease. It is characterized by wasting of the muscles (muscular dystrophy), cataracts, heart conduction defects, endocrine changes, and myotonia. Myotonic dystrophy can occur in patients of any age.
Noonan syndrome	Noonan Syndrome is a relatively common autosomal dominant congenital disorder considered to be a type of dwarfism, that affects both males and females equally. It used to be referred to as the male version of Turner's syndrome (and is still sometimes described in this way); however, the genetic causes of Noonan syndrome and Turner syndrome are distinct. The principal features include congenital heart defect, short stature, learning problems, pectus excavatum, impaired blood clotting, and a characteristic configuration of facial features including a webbed neck.
Orchitis	Orchitis is a condition of the testes involving inflammation. It can also involve swelling and frequent infection. Symptoms Symptoms of orchitis are similar to those of testicular torsion.

Anejaculation	Anejaculation is the pathological inability to ejaculate in males, with (orgasmic) or without (anorgasmic) orgasm. It can depend on one or more of several causes, including (ordered by frequency)': • Sexual inhibition • Pharmacological inhibition • Autonomic nervous system malfunction • Prostatectomy - surgical removal of the prostate. • Ejaculatory duct obstruction Anejaculation, especially the orgasmic variant, is usually indistinguishable from retrograde ejaculation. However, a negative urinalysis measuring no abnormal presence of spermatozoa in the urine will eliminate a retrograde ejaculation diagnosis.
Vas deferens	The vas deferens, also called ductus deferens is part of the male anatomy of many vertebrates; they transport sperm from the epididymis in anticipation of ejaculation. Structure There are two ducts, connecting the left and right epididymis to the ejaculatory ducts in order to move sperm. Each tube is about 30 centimeters long (in humans) and is muscular (surrounded by smooth muscle).
Vasectomy	Vasectomy is a surgical procedure in which the vasa deferentia of a man are severed, and sometimes tied or sealed. Procedure

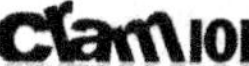

Usually done in an outpatient setting, a traditional vasectomy involves numbing of the scrotum with local anesthetic after which one or two small incisions are made, allowing a surgeon to gain access to the vas deferens of each testicle. The vasa deferentia are cut and sometimes sealed by ligating, cauterizing, or clamping.

Vasectomy reversal

Vasectomy reversal is a term used for surgical procedures that reconnect the male reproductive tract after interruption by a vasectomy. Two procedures are possible at the time of vasectomy reversal: vasovasostomy (vas deferens to vas deferens connection) and vasoepididymostomy (epididymis to vas deferens connection). Although vasectomy is considered a permanent form of contraception, advances in microsurgery have improved the success of vasectomy reversal procedures.

Microsurgery

Microsurgery is a general term for surgery requiring an operating microscope. The most obvious developments have been procedures developed to allow anastomosis of successively smaller blood vessels and nerves (typically 1 mm in diameter) which have allowed transfer of tissue from one part of the body to another and re-attachment of severed parts. Although microsurgery is used mostly in plastic surgery, microsurgical techniques are utilized by all specialties today, especially those involved in reconstructive surgery such as: general surgery, ophthalmology, orthopedic surgery, gynecological surgery, otolaryngology, neurosurgery, oral and maxillofacial surgery, and pediatric surgery.

Vasovasostomy

Vasovasostomy is a surgery by which vasectomies are partially reversed. Another surgery for vasectomy reversal is vasoepididymostomy.

History

Vasovasostomy is a form of microsurgery first performed by Earl Owen in 1971.

Electroejaculation

Electroejaculation is a procedure used to obtain semen samples from sexually mature male mammals. The procedure is applied for breeding programs and research purposes in various species, as well as in the treatment of an ejaculatory dysfunction in human males.

Electroejaculation is usually carried out under a general anesthetic.

Ejaculatory duct

The ejaculatory ducts (ductus ejaculatorii) are paired structures in male anatomy, about 2 cm in length.

Each ejaculatory duct is formed by the union of the vas deferens with the duct of the seminal vesicle. They pass through the prostate, and empty into the urethra at the Colliculus seminalis.

Ejaculatory duct

The ejaculatory ducts (ductus ejaculatorii) are paired structures in male anatomy, about 2 cm in length.

Each ejaculatory duct is formed by the union of the vas deferens with the duct of the seminal vesicle. They pass through the prostate, and empty into the urethra at the Colliculus seminalis.

Citrate

A citrate can refer either to the conjugate base of citric acid, ($C_3H_5O(COO)_3^{3-}$), or to the esters of citric acid. An example of the former, a salt is trisodium citrate; an ester is triethyl citrate.

Other citric acid ions

Since citric acid is a multifunctional acid, intermediate ions exist, hydrogen citrate ion, $HC_6H_5O_7^{2-}$ and dihydrogen citrate ion, $H_2C_6H_5O_7^{-}$.

Antineoplastic

Antineoplastic drugs inhibit and combat the development of cancer.

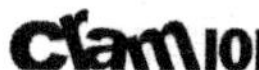

In the Anatomical Therapeutic Chemical Classification System, they are classified under L01.

Modes of action

There are many classes of antineoplastics:

- Alkylating agents
- Antimetabolites
- Antimitotics like Taxol: bind to tubulin and microtubules to inhibit spindle dynamics and thus block cell division
- Topoisomerase II inhibitors, stopping DNA from being unwound, which is required for both DNA replication and RNA/protein synthesis.
- Generating free radicals.

Examples

- taxanes
    - paclitaxel (Taxol).
    - docetaxel (Taxotere).
- actinomycin (L01DA01).

Insemination

Insemination is the introduction of sperm into the female uterus of a mammal or the oviduct of an oviparous (egg-laying) animal. There are however less conventional means of introduction of the sperms, for example, the sperms can be introduced violently by traumatic insemination, parenteral injection through the body wall, such as in some species of Hemiptera. In some species of animals, the sperms find their way through the body wall when the spermatophore is left in contact with the female's skin, such as in the Onychophora.

Intracytoplasmic sperm injection

Intracytoplasmic sperm injection is an in vitro fertilization procedure in which a single sperm is injected directly into an egg.

Indications

	This procedure is most commonly used to overcome male infertility problems, although it may also be used where eggs cannot easily be penetrated by sperm, and occasionally as a method of in vitro fertilization, especially that associated with sperm donation. It can be used in teratozoospermia.
Preimplantation genetic diagnosis	In medicine and (clinical) genetics pre-implantation genetic diagnosis (Preimplantation genetic diagnosis or PIGD) (also known as embryo screening) refers to procedures that are performed on embryos prior to implantation, sometimes even on oocytes prior to fertilization. Preimplantation genetic diagnosis is considered another way to prenatal diagnosis. Its main advantage is that it avoids selective pregnancy termination as the method makes it highly likely that the baby will be free of the disease under consideration.
Semen quality	Semen quality is a measure of the ability of semen to accomplish fertilization. Thus, it is a measure of fertility in a man. It is the sperm in the semen that are of importance, and therefore semen quality involves both sperm quantity and quality.
Fertility	Fertility is the natural capability of giving life. As a measure, "fertility rate" is the number of children born per couple, person or population. Fertility differs from fecundity, which is defined as the potential for reproduction (influenced by gamete production, fertilisation and carrying a pregnancy to term).
Mutation	In molecular biology and genetics, mutations are changes in a genomic sequence: the DNA sequence of a cell's genome or the DNA or RNA sequence of a virus. Mutations are caused by radiation, viruses, transposons and mutagenic chemicals, as well as errors that occur during meiosis or DNA replication. They can also be induced by the organism itself, by cellular processes such as hypermutation.
Formulation	A formulation is a mixture that is prepared according to a specific procedure (called a "formula"). Formulations are made for particular applications and normally are more effective than their individual components when these are used singly. Formulations are commercially produced for drugs, cosmetics, coatings, cleaning agents, foods, paints, pesticides and many other products.

Dihydrotestosterone	Dihydrotestosterone is an androgen, synthesized primarily in the prostate gland, testes, hair follicles, and adrenal glands by the enzyme 5α-reductase by means of reducing the 4,5 double-bond of the hormone testosterone. Effects on sexual development In men, approximately 5% of testosterone undergoes 5α-reduction to form the more potent androgen, dihydrotestosterone. DHT has three times greater affinity for androgen receptors than testosterone and has 15-30 times greater affinity than adrenal androgens.
Dehydroepiandrosterone	5-Dehydroepiandrosterone is a 19-carbon endogenous natural steroid hormone. It is the major secretory steroidal product of the adrenal glands and is also produced by the gonads and the brain. DHEA is the most abundant circulating steroid in humans.
Hematology	Hematology, also spelled haematology, is the branch of internal medicine, physiology, pathology, clinical laboratory work, and pediatrics that is concerned with the study of blood, the blood-forming organs, and blood diseases. Hematology includes the study of etiology, diagnosis, treatment, prognosis, and prevention of blood diseases. The laboratory work that goes into the study of blood is frequently performed by a medical technologist.
Adrenal gland	In mammals, the adrenal glands (also known as suprarenal glands) are endocrine glands that sit on top of the kidneys; in humans, the right suprarenal gland is triangular shaped while the left suprarenal gland is semilunar shaped. They are chiefly responsible for releasing hormones in conjunction with stress through the synthesis of corticosteroids such as cortisol and catecholamines, such as epinephrine. Adrenal glands affect kidney function through the secretion of aldosterone, a hormone involved in regulating plasma osmolarity.
Cerebrospinal fluid	Cerebrospinal fluid Liquor cerebrospinalis, is a clear, colorless bodily fluid, that occupies the subarachnoid space and the ventricular system around and inside the brain and spinal cord. In essence, the brain "floats" in it. The CSF occupies the space between the arachnoid mater (the middle layer of the brain cover, meninges), and the pia mater (the layer of the meninges closest to the brain).

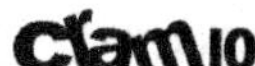

Hydronephrosis	Hydronephrosis is distension and dilation of the renal pelvis calyces, usually caused by obstruction of the free flow of urine from the kidney, leading to progressive atrophy of the kidney. In cases of hydroureteronephrosis, there is distention of both the ureter and the renal pelvis and calices. Signs and symptoms The signs and symptoms of hydronephrosis depend upon whether the obstruction is acute or chronic, partial or complete, unilateral or bilateral.
Ureter	In human anatomy, the ureters are muscular tubes that propel urine from the kidneys to the urinary bladder. In the adult, the ureters are usually 25-30 cm (10-12 in) long and ~3-4 mm in diameter. In humans, the ureters arise from the renal pelvis on the medial aspect of each kidney before descending towards the bladder on the front of the psoas major muscle.
Percutaneous nephrolithotomy	Percutaneous nephrolithotomy is a surgical procedure to remove stones from the kidney by a small puncture wound (up to about 1 cm) through the skin. It is most suitable to remove stones of more than 2 cm in size. It is usually done under general anesthesia or spinal anesthesia.
Granuloma	Granuloma is a medical term for a roughly spherical mass of immune cells that forms when the immune system attempts to wall off substances that it perceives as foreign but is unable to eliminate. Such substances include infectious organisms such as bacteria and fungi as well as other materials such as keratin and suture fragments. A granuloma is therefore a special type of inflammation that can occur in a wide variety of diseases.
Granuloma inguinale	Granuloma inguinale is a bacterial disease characterized by ulcerative genital lesions that is endemic in many less developed regions. It is also known as donovanosis, granuloma genitoinguinale, granuloma inguinale tropicum, granuloma venereum, granuloma venereum genitoinguinale, lupoid form of groin ulceration, serpiginous ulceration of the groin, ulcerating granuloma of the pudendum and ulcerating sclerosing granuloma. The disease often goes untreated because of the scarcity of medical treatment in the countries in which it is found.

CPSIA information can be obtained at www.ICGtesting.com
Printed in the USA
LVOW03s1613231214

420148LV00001B/44/P